YANG SHENG

This book is dedicated
to my mother.

YANG SHENG

THE ART OF CHINESE SELF-HEALING

KATIE BRINDLE

Hardie Grant
BOOKS

CONTENTS

INTRODUCTION

'A drop of prevention is better than a bucketload of cure.'
ANCIENT CHINESE PROVERB

Yang sheng may be the most important concept in Chinese medicine you've never heard of. The direct translation is 'nourish life'. To explain a bit more fully, yang sheng will help you balance your whole self for a long, wise and happy life.

Sounds like a big promise? You might think it's even bigger when I tell you that yang sheng is the self-care part of Chinese medicine – a self-healing system – which means you can do all the treatments yourself, most of them completely for free, putting yourself in the driving seat of your health.

BETTER ENERGY, SLEEP & MOOD

It's my dream to help people discover yang sheng techniques. These simple but powerful habit and lifestyle changes have transformed my life. I know the knowledge in this book can do the same for you. Living the yang sheng way will improve the way you feel in so many ways, from your sleep and digestion, to your skin and energy levels. Yang sheng has mood benefits, too: getting into balance will bring you closer to a default state of calm and quiet contentment. And you can get all of these benefits in just a few minutes a day.

This book will explain the principles of yang sheng, which is currently relatively unknown in the West. But, most importantly, it will show you how to fit this system into your life, easily and effortlessly. You can use the book as the beginning of a journey deep into Chinese medicine or you can simply add a few of the suggestions to your daily routine.

Chinese medicine is ancient, yet it's still relevant today. It has helped millions of people and it can help you, too. Life has evolved, but the mechanisms of our body haven't really changed. The actual techniques have stood the test of thousands of years. What I have tried to do is to bring them up to date with a modern format and instructions. I only ask that you keep an open mind and give it a try.

BENEFITS OF DAILY HEALTH MAINTENANCE

Yang sheng has such a different way of thinking about the body, but this is precisely why it's valuable. Western medicine tends not to focus on disease prevention. We, in turn, take our good health for granted until we're ill; at which point, we treat the symptoms collectively rather than looking for a root cause.

If you fell sick in ancient China, it was regarded as a failure of preventative medicine. The principle of yang sheng – and indeed of Chinese medicine – is that if you eliminate small health niggles as they arise, you'll prevent bigger ones happening. There's an ancient Chinese proverb: 'Waiting to treat illnesses after they manifest is like waiting to dig a well after one is thirsty.'

When you adopt yang sheng as a daily practice, you are being proactive about your health maintenance, using what I consider to be the most powerful and time-tested of techniques. Think of it like this: regular yang sheng will do for your wellbeing what tooth brushing does for your mouth. You wouldn't dream of not brushing your teeth each day – and once you see and feel the benefits of yang sheng, you will want to continue doing it every day, too. It is daily maintenance for your body, mind and spirit.

ARE YOU IN BALANCE?

Chinese medicine has a sophisticated understanding of how the body works physically, emotionally and spiritually, but also energetically, because it says you are all of those things wrapped up together.

The philosophy is that any disease starts with a disruption of energy flow, which happens before you notice any symptoms. The good news is, you can treat those subtle energetic imbalances before they progress and cause obvious physical symptoms. As strange as this may sound, I have seen in practice that it really works.

A disruption of energy flow can manifest in all kinds of ways before you become ill. For example, are you sleeping well? You may not be a hardcore insomniac, but do you wake up exhausted? You may not be sick, but are you quite well every day? Do you feel strong? Are you calm? Do you bounce out of bed ready for action? Sadly, most of us feel under par at least some of the time. Our modern lifestyle leaves us as out of balance as a single person on a seesaw.

Maybe that's why you've picked up this book – you don't feel quite right but you can't put your finger on a cause. My patients often come to me because of poor sleep, low energy, depression or chronic pain. These are all conditions Western medicine can't resolve easily, but which have left them desperate to find a solution.

I often see patients suffering from low libido, too. Sex is often a casualty of modern living. Think about it like this: you can live without your fertility, so it's usually the first bodily system to get shut down when the body is stressed and needs to conserve resources. Which, given how life-affirming sex can be, is a huge pity.

The more symptoms of ill health you have, the more out of balance Chinese medicine will assess you to be. You don't have to understand exactly how and where you are out of balance to get yourself back into alignment – another of the joys of Chinese medicine. You just have to learn and understand a few of the *right* things – then do them.

Good health is not something you achieve with an hour a day in the gym (although exercise has its place) or by depriving yourself of your most-loved indulgences. Rather, health is something to nurture with a series of little moments, the yang sheng techniques I'll be showing you, throughout the day.

LESS IS DEFINITELY MORE

I'd say most of my clients are probably doing too much. You know yourself when you're doing too much worrying, too much work, too much socialising. According to Chinese medicine, less can be more. Sometimes, you may be delighted to hear, a nap is better than a workout. You can actually over-exercise and have too many rules about what you're eating and which foods you are giving up.

Often, people come into the clinic having changed their diet and started taking supplements, but they still feel exhausted or anxious. As I explain to them, it's because they don't have the full picture of what it takes to nurture their health. Yang sheng is the full picture. Yes, food and digestion are important but so is the right kind of breathing and exercise, self-massage and looking after your emotions and spirit, too. Once you have all these elements in place, you'll be in balance. And then there will be no need to ban the small things that sweeten life – such as the morning coffee you treasure or the glass or two of red after a tough day.

That said, when you try yang sheng, you'll notice life begins to go a little more smoothly. There will be more good days. Even better, you'll want to adopt yang sheng techniques because they are, in themselves, pleasurable. It's time to take steps to look after you.

WHERE YANG SHENG COMES FROM

Most likely what you already know of Chinese medicine is herbs and acupuncture, but there is so, so much more this ancient wisdom can teach us about nurturing the body, mind and spirit to be in harmony with natural rhythms and universal laws.

So why aren't we all using yang sheng already? It comes from classical Chinese medicine, which has a history of over 5,000 years. However, after the People's Republic of China was established in 1949, the landscape of health care in China shifted dramatically and much of its knowledge barely survived. While the new Ministry of Health paid attention to the practical side of Chinese medicine such as acupuncture and herbal medicines to treat disease, classical Chinese medicine was widely ignored.

Luckily for us, the political fashions shifted, and during the 1980s many of the traditional classical Chinese medicine texts were republished. Since then, interest in the original form has been steadily growing, both in China and abroad.

The *Huangdi Neijing* is classical Chinese medicine's most famous medical textbook, thought to be between 4,000 and 5,000 years old. Even now, this fully comprehensive tome on health, lifestyle and medical advice is so relevant, underlining the importance of how you sleep, eat, work and exercise, as well as how your emotions relate to physical health. All Chinese medicine can be traced back to the

Neijing but, in reality, by the time it was written these self-healing techniques had already been developed and refined over thousands of years.

Most of the techniques in this book come from this ancient Chinese wisdom. This means they are owned by no one. So, just as with chicken soup recipes, there are endless variations. I've tried to keep my version true to the spirit of Chinese medicine. At the same time, I've distilled it so it's easy to understand, to make it easy for you to fully steep your modern life in this life-changing and ancient wisdom.

I'm so happy to be sharing this small part of the priceless treasure chest of Chinese medicine. I know that once you start to feel the profound upswing in your energy levels and the inner calm and increased wellbeing that comes from practising yang sheng, you'll want to do more.

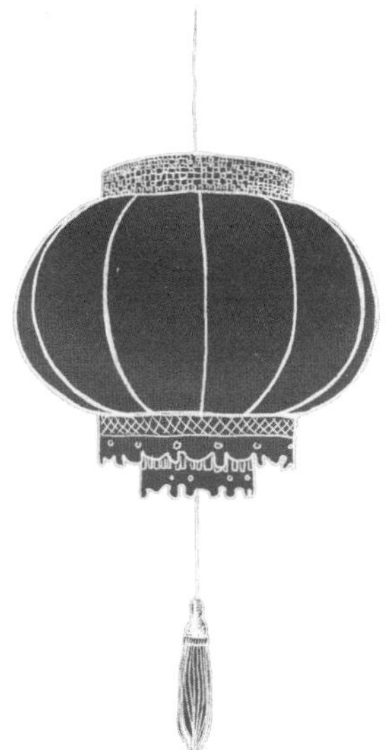

HOW I DISCOVERED YANG SHENG

My journey to Chinese medicine started after a car accident in my early 20s. The whiplash I sustained affected my vocal cords, abruptly ending my dreams of becoming an opera singer. Even a year after the accident, I was still in constant pain. I was unhappy, too, having had to give up on singing; my passion.

After much trial and error of various therapies, I finally found something that helped; Chinese medicine, in the form of acupuncture and a kind of massage called tui na.

I was amazed at how, with the right kind of help, my body was able to heal itself. In a matter of months, my neck was pain-free, although it's always the telltale place that is first to suffer when I get out of balance.

As my physical pain receded, so did my emotional pain. I decided that my mission in life would be to learn how to help others, using this remarkable healing system. Soon after, I trained in massage and reflexology. It was a few years later, while I was qualifying as a Five Elements Chinese medical practitioner from the UK's College of Integrated Chinese Medicine, that I first heard of yang sheng. Now, with my patients, I specialise in a combination of detailed diagnosis and self-treatment, drawing upon the extraordinary legacy of yang sheng.

Don't get me wrong, I'm not at all against Western medical expertise. I appreciate what it does and has done for me and millions of others, but it's fair to say there's a gap that medicine doesn't address and that's the 'almost-well', the 'not feeling so good', the tired out and over-stressed. This is a gap I have seen Chinese medicine – specifically yang sheng – fill beautifully.

I have drawn upon the system's remarkable heritage to make these ancient techniques achievable and accessible, a way to self-care, if you like. I am in no way a master of Chinese medicine. I'm, like you – in the trenches, living my modern lifestyle, being imperfect. What I hope is that the tools that changed my life and those of many others can help you feel energised, well and healthy, too.

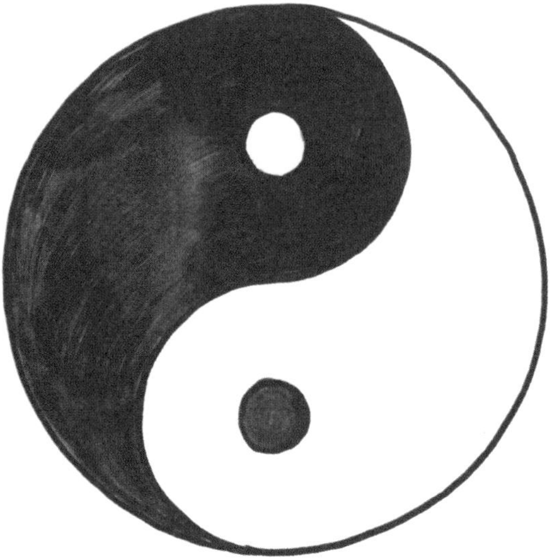

HOW TO USE THIS BOOK

To most people, Chinese medicine is complex and unfamiliar – I hope to make it clear and doable. Although it's difficult to translate, it can be reduced to some simple truths. We may each be unique, but our bodies share patterns of behaviour.

At the end of the first section you'll find three key yang sheng techniques. If you want to start practising now, these are ideal. Not only are they super quick but, hopefully, how you feel will inspire you to try more.

The book is filled with practical, self-healing rituals you can pick and choose to fit easily into your daily routine. In the second section, you'll find chapters dealing with specific areas from digestion to sleep to your emotions, along with simple techniques to support balance and good health. Due to the holistic nature of Chinese medicine, they will all improve your general wellbeing, too.

In the third section, you'll learn why living with the seasons is so important to Chinese medicine and your health. Starting with the season you're in right now, I suggest you make a few small changes to adapt and align with nature.

Throughout the book I'll refer to certain key concepts in Chinese medicine. So, we'll start with a short (and I hope clear!) explanation of each. You don't need to know all of this for the techniques to work, so you can come back to this section if you'd prefer.

Let's get started.

PART 1

KEY PRINCIPLES

IDEAS FROM CHINESE MEDICINE

'The journey of a thousand miles begins with one step.'
LAO TZU

TAOISM

Taoism is a Chinese philosophy and science of life that dates back over 5,000 years. It is the philosophical basis of Chinese medicine.

The word 'Tao' means 'the way' – the way of nature and the universe. Taoism is about understanding that your body, mind and spirit all impact each other – and the universe.

You could think of it like this: everything in the universe comprises of qi. Qi has its own explanation on page 23, but its most simple translation is 'life energy'. As part of the universe, we too are comprised of energy and this is what connects us inherently to everything around us. And Chinese medicine treats the human body as a small universe, with our emotions, energy and internal organs all connecting and in relationship with each other.

To be a Taoist is to work out how best to live considering your own nature and your environment. It suggests lifestyle habits to encourage a long and healthy journey through life. Taoism prescribes that if you live in harmony with the energies of the planet and seasons, you will thrive.

YIN AND YANG

Yin and yang represents harmony and balance. It says that everything in the universe – including your body and your health – is made up of two opposing forces that are in a constant state of change.

If yin is a negative force, yang is positive. While yin is feminine, yang is masculine. Yin is passive and slow, yang is active and fast.

Even though they are opposite, yin and yang cannot exist without each other. For optimum health, they should be roughly equal, both in your body and your life.

To find that balance, look at what is yin and what is yang about you. A lot of modern imbalance comes from the fact that the world is now so yang: fast, aggressive, active. So, one of the main things you'll do throughout the book is learn how to nurture your yin and get more passive, nourishing energy into your life.

By the very nature of being human, our lives will always create imbalance. Symptoms, while unpleasant, are not the problem – they are alerts, signalling that your yin and yang are out of balance. The worse your symptoms, the more out of balance you are.

You don't need to make massive adjustments. Start with the small changes offered by the yang sheng techniques, even if you just do one minute at a time. More than ever, we need these techniques to carve out moments of calm throughout the day. Think of each one as a quick reset for your yin and yang energies.

Yin and yang is one of the universal rules that apply to all of nature – including us. As we are fundamentally connected to nature, synching with it is the best way to balance your yin and yang. This is why yang sheng prescribes that living in harmony with nature is so important.

This may all sound quite unfamiliar, but once you start to apply the theory in practical ways, you will quickly see a difference.

QI

Qi is explained in many different ways, but most commonly as energy or life force. Qi is the living vibration and the basis for all that exists. It is the energy that flows inside all of us and through every living object on the planet. Think of every one of us as little ecosystems within a bigger one.

Even when you sit completely still, there will be some movement happening inside you. Your organs, your heart beating, fluids moving – every cell is constantly in motion. All these different types of energy combined with your breath is what makes up your qi.

A good explanation for qi that I've heard is this: imagine yourself as a wave. You are, at the same time, an individual wave and a part of the ocean. Your qi is yours, but you share it with the planet.

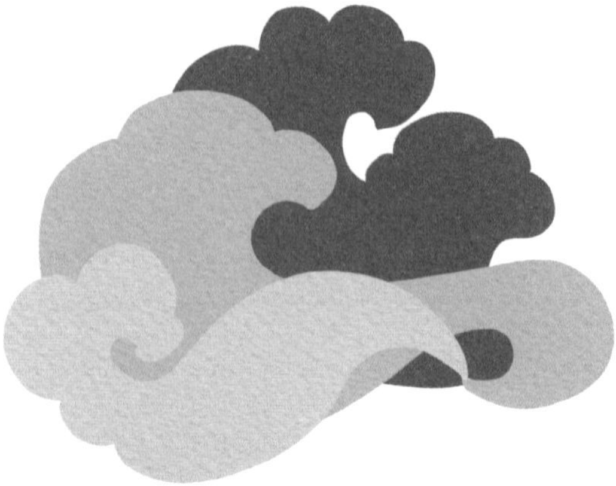

Qi isn't the same as the circulation, but it is linked. When you stimulate your blood flow or move your lymphatic fluid, your qi is also stimulated. Everything flows together.

The channels in which qi flows are called meridians. They travel up the front of the body and down the back of it (see opposite for a simplified diagram). According to Chinese medicine, the quality and movement of qi through the body determines your health. The ideal state is one of smooth flow with no imbalances or blockages, which are called stagnation or stagnant qi. If you have continued stagnation, whether physical, emotional or spiritual, Chinese medicine says this will eventually manifest as disease.

Along the meridians are places where qi is more abundant and behaves in a way that makes it accessible; these are where acupuncture needles are inserted. Each point will have a particular function related to the mind, body or spirit, or a combination.

There are other ways besides acupuncture that you can stimulate these points and so encourage the free flow

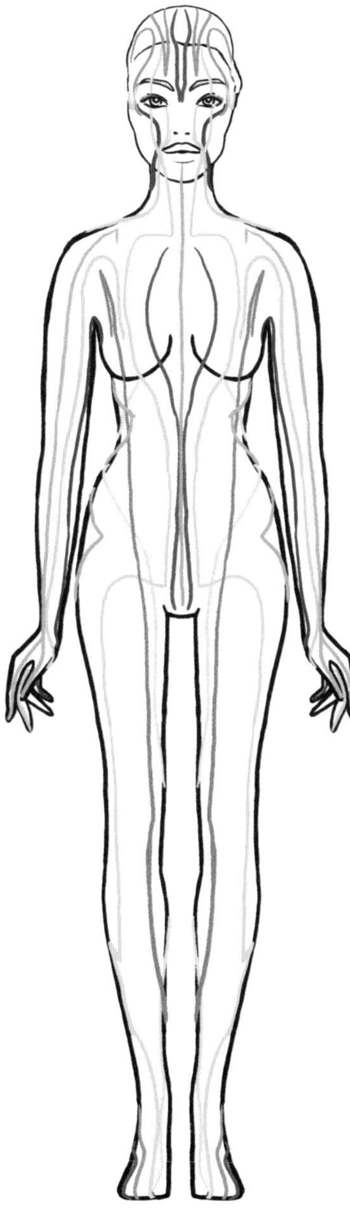

of qi. There is acupressure and tui na, both types of massage, and another massage technique called gua sha (see page 31). There's also qigong, a system of exercise that manipulates the flow of qi using movement and breath (see page 27).

If you expend more qi than you acquire, you'll start to experience fatigue and other low-level health problems. The yang sheng techniques in this book are very much concerned with nurturing and boosting your qi and encouraging its smooth flow around the body. Build up your qi this way, and soon you'll feel it reflected in your energy, vigour and lust for life.

A word on inflammation: Triggered by our immune system, inflammation is crucial to fight infection or protect damaged tissue and heal wounds. It's a useful mechanism in the body's defences – until it goes into overdrive. Excessive chronic inflammation is increasingly seen by doctors as a key factor behind a great many diseases and health issues.

The rough equivalent of inflammation in Chinese medicine is called 'heat', although this is an over-simplification. For the purposes of this book, when I talk about clearing heat, I mean anti-inflammatory techniques. Qigong, for example, has been shown to reduce inflammation, as have many other mind-body techniques such as breathing and meditation. This, I believe, is where the healing power of yang sheng comes from.

KEY YANG SHENG TECHNIQUES

Qigong

There are a large variety of incredibly effective yang sheng techniques to choose from, including: being in nature, eating, exercise, sleep, sex, dance, music and the cultivation of the spirit, to name but a few. In this book we'll explore some of the ones I recommend most often in clinic.

Qigong, often called dynamic meditation, sits alongside gua sha (see page 31) as one of the self-healing pillars of Chinese medicine. Traditionally, it was used to prevent illness and to promote longevity as well as for spiritual enlightenment.

A martial art that's been practised for thousands of years in various forms, it's made up of sequences of flowing movements where the body, mind and breath are coordinated and relaxed. It looks similar to tai chi, as they have shared roots and work on the same principles.

The word 'qigong' translates as 'vital energy cultivation' – and this is what it does. While it physically works your body, it calms your mind and elevates your spirit. It is a perfect mixture of yin and yang, yin being the meditative part and yang the doing part, the movement.

Qigong is low impact; because of this, it has mostly been adopted by the older generation in the West. But everyone, young or old, will benefit hugely from how it builds strength and resilience and encourages the free flow of qi and blood around the body.

In studies, regular sessions of qigong have been shown to calm the stress response and promote relaxation, making it useful for pretty much everyone. In fact, it's as if qigong was invented for modern day health issues; research suggests it's helpful for conditions including anxiety, depression and high blood pressure as well as for bone health. There's also evidence qigong may improve immune function as well as reduce inflammation. In fact, its effects are simply remarkable.

Qigong is simple to practise at home – or, indeed, anywhere – as the basic movements are gentle on the body and super easy. But what I really love about it, is how you feel the meditative and energetic benefits so quickly. Doing it is so pleasurable – I can only describe the feeling as like spring water flowing through your body – yet it has such a remarkable impact on your long-term health.

BREATHING

In Chinese medicine, the importance of breathing good-quality air and breathing properly are key. The breath is one of the two ways you create qi (the other is eating and drinking). Breathing deeply – as you will be doing a lot with this technique – immediately relaxes the body because it stimulates the vagus nerve, which runs from the neck to the abdomen and is in charge of turning off the 'fight or flight' reflex. There is also evidence that stimulating the vagus nerve combats inflammation, so breathing properly will give you both instant and long-term benefits.

TAPPING

I'm a huge advocate of tapping, also called drumming. It's exactly what it says: tapping your body with a loose fist. If you do it with vigour, it stimulates your circulation, giving you an instant hit of invigoration. If you do it gently and slowly, you'll find it very relaxing. Studies show it may have great after effects on both mental health and immunity. In fact, it's even been called 'stem cell qigong' by Mantak Chia, a Taoist master.

> 'More than 5,000 years (ago) the Taoist masters discovered that our body has a marvellous regenerating, repairing and rebuilding power. By gently and gradually applying hitting on the body parts and vital organs, the old, sick and damaged cells will be completely broken up. The body sends its own stem cells to repair and regenerate the skin, organs, glands and all the body parts.' Master Mantak Chia.

Tapping is the basis of another technique – Emotional Freedom Technique, or EFT, currently a buzzword in health and wellness. In fact, the healing concepts on which EFT is based have been practised in Chinese medicine for over 5,000 years. Just as in acupuncture and acupressure, tapping on specific points along the meridian channels is said to restore a good flow of qi.

BAMBOO TAPPING

This is another way to tap, using a tool that looks like a long brush but with very hard and twangy bristles made of thin bamboo rods (or sometimes metal). It's a bit stronger than using your fingers – and it feels incredible. It may look a little unconventional, but the bamboo rods relieve stress in muscles, work to unblock the meridians and stimulate lymphatic drainage, making it highly beneficial. Follow the same routine as for tapping, but use the bamboo tapper instead of your fist.

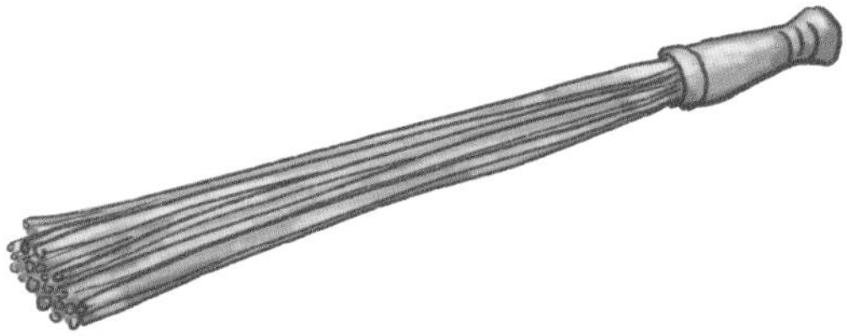

SHAKING

This is the simplest and most brilliant energiser, which involves simply shaking your entire body. Shaking gives your circulation an immediate kick start – it gets your blood and qi flowing and dislodges stagnation, so it's great in the morning, or as a pick me up if you are feeling sluggish. It's also good after a bad experience: animals and humans alike shake as a spontaneous self-healing response to trauma or shock. Think of it like pressing an emotional reset button.

Acupressure

Often described as 'acupuncture without the needles', acupressure involves stimulating points on or along the whole length of your meridian channels with a finger or jade tool, in order to release blocks. It helps to restore the flow of qi.

Gua sha

Gua sha is a type of therapeutic massage technique that you can do on yourself using a round-edged tool. It's been widely practised in China for thousands of years. 'Gua' means to scrape or rub, whilst 'sha' describes the temporary redness that results.

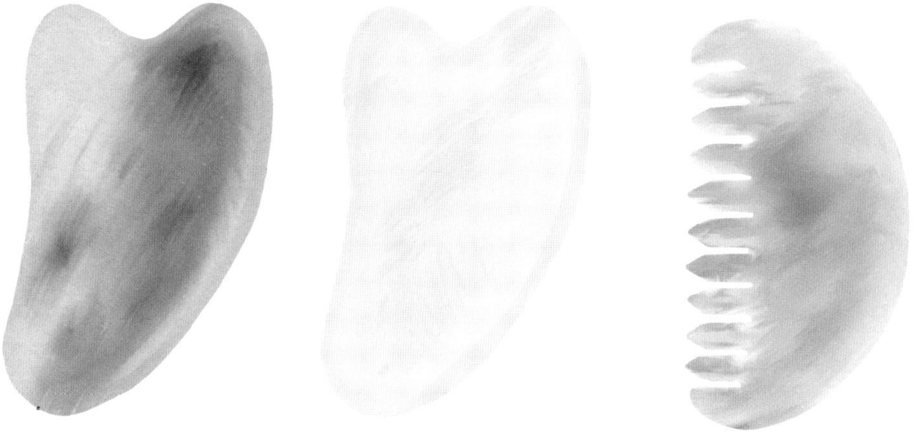

The principle is to press-stroke the skin until a red rash appears – hence the name. Possibly the redness is why gua sha hasn't been imported to the West before now. I assume people find it off putting, although the marks do fade fast. The healing principle behind gua sha is the same as that of cupping – you might remember the negative press coverage around Gwyneth Paltrow's cupping marks? More recently, those tell-tale circular marks have also been spotted on Andy Murray, Amir Khan and Michael Phelps; top athletes whose entire careers rest upon keeping themselves in peak condition.

What I find interesting is that every treatment you do is different. Gua sha is about clearing heat – or inflammation – out of your body, so the amount of sha that shows up will depend on the amount of heat you have.

Initial research suggests that gua sha offers anti-inflammatory and immune-boosting properties, although why is still not scientifically clear. Modern studies show gua sha increases blood flow to the surface of the skin. This helps boost the skin's circulation, bringing nutrients to the skin and boosting the lymphatic system, crucial for waste disposal and immunity. Regular gua sha has also been shown in studies to relieve muscular tension and may be helpful for improving sleep too.

FACIAL GUA SHA

Facial gua sha really is a game changer and many of my clients tell me how much they love the way it has transformed their skin. It's often the first yang sheng technique that people adopt, because you tend to see visible results quickly.

It's usually done with a jade or other crystal tool shaped like a half moon, so it can follow the contours of your face. However, you don't need the specialist tool, you can even use a Chinese porcelain soup spoon or a jam jar lid. If you are worried about redness, just practise before bed and go slowly to start with.

The boost to your microcirculation during gua sha floods the skin with fresh nutrients, over time boosting levels of collagen and elastin. Done regularly, it smooths and plumps the skin, reducing the appearance of fine lines and wrinkles.

Also, gua sha is great for reducing morning puffiness and congestion, by gently encouraging the movement of lymphatic fluid, which can't flow by itself. It only moves when we move – or when we move it. Gua sha releases tension in facial muscles and soothes sore eyes and skin, making your complexion look brighter and generally more radiant.

You'd be surprised at how much tension you store in and among the 43 muscles of the face. Using a gua sha tool allows you to work deeper into the muscles and fascia than by using fingers alone, so you can consciously release where you are knotted or tight. Finally, facial gua sha activates acupressure points along the 12 major meridian lines in your face.

BODY GUA SHA

The body gua sha tool is also a half-moon shape but is made of thinner jade or metal, because your body benefits from a little more intensity. You can also use a jam-jar lid.

Gua sha was traditionally given by family members or friends for a huge range of conditions, from fever, muscle pain and musculoskeletal problems to inflammation, chronic coughs, sinusitis, diarrhoea and migraines. It was also considered good for the prevention of illness, with treatment focussed on a particular area of the body depending on the issue. It's said to maintain and strengthen your constitution, increasing your longevity.

As part of yang sheng, we use it to stay well and keep the body and emotions balanced. That's because after gua sha on the body, most people report feeling better both physically and emotionally, with a feeling of weightlessness and relief. Chinese medicine explains it like this: emotions and consciousness are stored in the organs, so when emotions and thoughts go unexpressed, the flow of qi in the body becomes stuck. This is felt as knots and adhesions, muscular pain and tightness. A healthy body and mind needs blood to move freely so thoughts and feelings can move freely through the consciousness. And gua sha helps this to happen.

COMBING THERAPY

All the body's meridians have either direct or indirect connections with somewhere on the head and scalp, so combing the head – usually with a jade or other crystal comb – stimulates them. It also increases circulation, delivering more nutrients to the hair follicle, which is reputed to promote hair growth. Best of all, and especially if you like your head being touched, head massage has been shown to be a speedy stress reliever.

Mineral bathing

The Chinese have known for centuries that bathing with aromatic ingredients and minerals alongside breathing techniques is a stress-killing combination. Only recently has science begun to understand how 'passive heating' – getting hot in a bath, shower or sauna – improves health by helping reduce chronic inflammation, improve cardiovascular health and regulate blood sugar levels.

In one of the traditional Chinese ways of bathing, you alternate two or three times between hot and cold water, exfoliating in the heat when your pores are open, following with cold water to close them (see Mineral Bath Ritual, page 82). Avoid extremes of temperature if you're not in good health, and particularly if you have high or low blood pressure, skin issues, or are pregnant.

Foot bathing

When I recommend bathing, some of my patients say, 'I don't own a bath!'. In fact, you don't need one. Foot bathing has a heritage and practice of its own in China, and all you need to get the benefits is a washing-up bowl. I love foot bathing – although it's simple and frugal, it feels supremely luxurious.

The feet have more than 60 acupuncture points each, corresponding to many parts and organs of the body. Chinese medicine says that when you soak the feet in warm water, the resulting slightly raised body temperature will unblock the meridians.

HEALING CRISIS

Chinese medicine invented the concept of the healing crisis, although it's been adopted by various forms of holistic therapies – you may have heard of it in homeopathy. It appears in the ancient text *Shangshu* (*The Book of Documents*), written over 2,000 years ago, and its Chinese name is the Ming Xuan reaction.

Chinese medicine explains that if toxicity is left to linger in the body's storage areas, it causes stagnant qi, which will eventually manifest in physical symptoms and disease. One of the basic principles of Chinese medicine is 'purge and nourish'. You clear out what you don't need, then nourish your body to support and strengthen it.

In practice, when people start doing yang sheng techniques, they sometimes feel worse before they feel better. This is an important part of the process; it is the body clearing itself in order to restore balance and a positive sign of returning to health. The best thing about a healing crisis? Not feeling great will force you to take time out to recuperate and regenerate. Don't soldier on, give in to it.

While the symptoms – headaches, sweating, cold-like symptoms – might make you think you're going down with a 'bug', there's one indication it's a healing crisis; you will want to sleep, a lot. (As a precaution, if your symptoms persist for longer than three days, see your GP.) If it happens to you, you need to do these three things:

- Let any treatment take its course. Don't try to suppress the symptoms with medication.
- Rest. This will allow the body to use its energy on healing.
- Make sure you stay hydrated.

As you are self-treating and not under the supervision of a practitioner, I'd like to stress the importance of introducing these techniques gradually, so as to soften any healing crisis you might experience. It will take longer, but your symptoms are likely to be less severe.

Three daily techniques to rebalance your body and mind

These techniques are a great place to start your yang sheng journey. Not only are they short but they're based on what you already do – breathing and moving – just upgraded. Together, they will help relax your body and, the Chinese would say, release stagnant qi and move your fluids. In Western terms, you'd say they boost your circulation including your lymphatic system. These techniques are so short that they're doable daily.

1. ONE-MINUTE RESCUE BREATH RITUAL

DO THIS AT LEAST ONCE A DAY

However busy you are, you have to breathe! While you may not have paid much attention to your breathing before, you'll discover it's the key to controlling your stress levels. When you're stressed, it greatly affects your digestive system, which is why focusing positive energy on this area is so beneficial. This effortless technique is powerful because it gives your mind something to focus on. It's basically a minute of easy meditation.

1 Start seated, lying down or standing; however you're comfortable. Breathe in through the nose then sharply out through the mouth, sticking out your tongue and making

a 'Haaaaa' noise as you do so. This clears the stale air that accumulates in your lungs when you breathe shallowly. Repeat three times.

2 With your eyes closed, breathe in for five counts through the nose and out for five counts through the nose. Think of inhaling the oxygen deeply, to fill your chest cavity and down to your abdomen. Let your focus descend to your lower abdomen; your heart rate will slow, your blood pressure will drop and your muscles will begin to relax. Don't worry about whether you're breathing right – the key is taking your focus down into your body.

3 Visualise a smile happening in your lower abdomen. Do this by recalling the warm feeling you get when you smile, then imagine sending that feeling to your lower stomach.

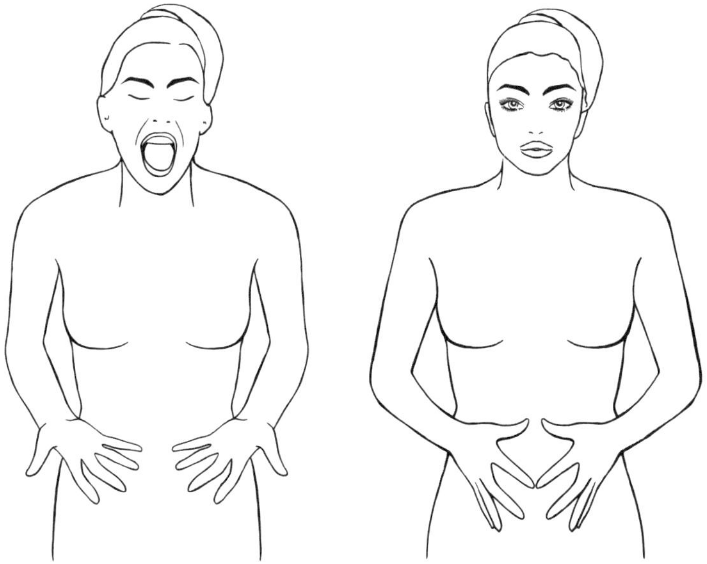

2. ONE-MINUTE TAPPING RITUAL

DO THIS AT LEAST ONCE A DAY

This exercise gives your circulation a serious wake-up call, so it's a great antidote to feeling tired or sluggish. Do it on waking then repeat regularly throughout the day; for example, every time you wash your hands. Tying it to a regular action will help you remember to do it.

1 With a loose fist or cupped hand, rapidly and firmly pat down the insides then up the outsides of the arms. Then, pat down the outsides and up the insides of the legs including onto the feet.
2 Pat in a circle around your abdomen, your lower back, all over your head and finally your thymus (between your breasts).

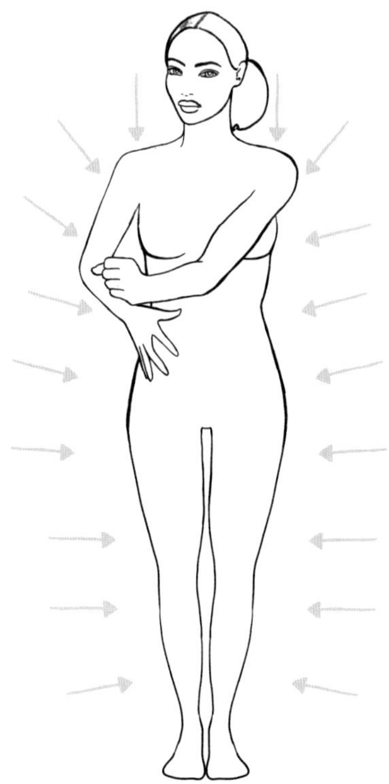

A word on other healing therapies: I love good treatments, and I work with some outstanding therapists. A great therapeutic relationship is a huge asset to your health, but not everyone is able to commit to regular treatments. If you can't, self-healing is a valuable alternative. If you can, use these techniques in between your sessions to amplify the benefits.

The importance of nature: Being in balance with and aligning to nature are fundamental to Taoism. I suggest one of the first changes you make is to get out into green spaces more. Immersing yourself in nature has a range of benefits, like supporting your immune system, reducing stress hormones and boosting creativity.

Stepping away from your screen and getting outside is about more than just fresh air, although that's good too. Your eyes naturally love to look at the shapes in nature, which have been proven to relax us. Seeing nature has also been shown to increase positive emotions, which boosts anti-inflammatory proteins called cytokines. Even a plant on your desk can be hugely beneficial.

3. LIFTING THE SKY

DO THIS AT LEAST ONCE A DAY

Like all qigong movements, there are lots of slightly different versions of this exercise. This is one of the simplest; it will engage most of your meridians (energy channels) as well as strengthen your abdominal muscles.

1 Start standing, feet shoulder width apart. Keep your eyes relaxed and half shut. Have your hands out in front at hip level, arms slightly bent, palms facing the floor with tips of fingers almost touching.
2 Breathe out, then engage your abdomen. Look at your hands.
3 Take a deep breath in and, as you do, press your hands towards the floor, then let them come up in a half circle, palms outwards. Follow your hands with your eyes. Keep your palms flat and your elbows slightly bent.
4 When your hands reach forehead level, push upwards, as though you are lifting the sky, looking up.
5 When your hands reach the top, breathe out as you separate your arms out to your sides and move them down in a circle. Let your arms and gaze drop back to centre. Repeat for one minute.

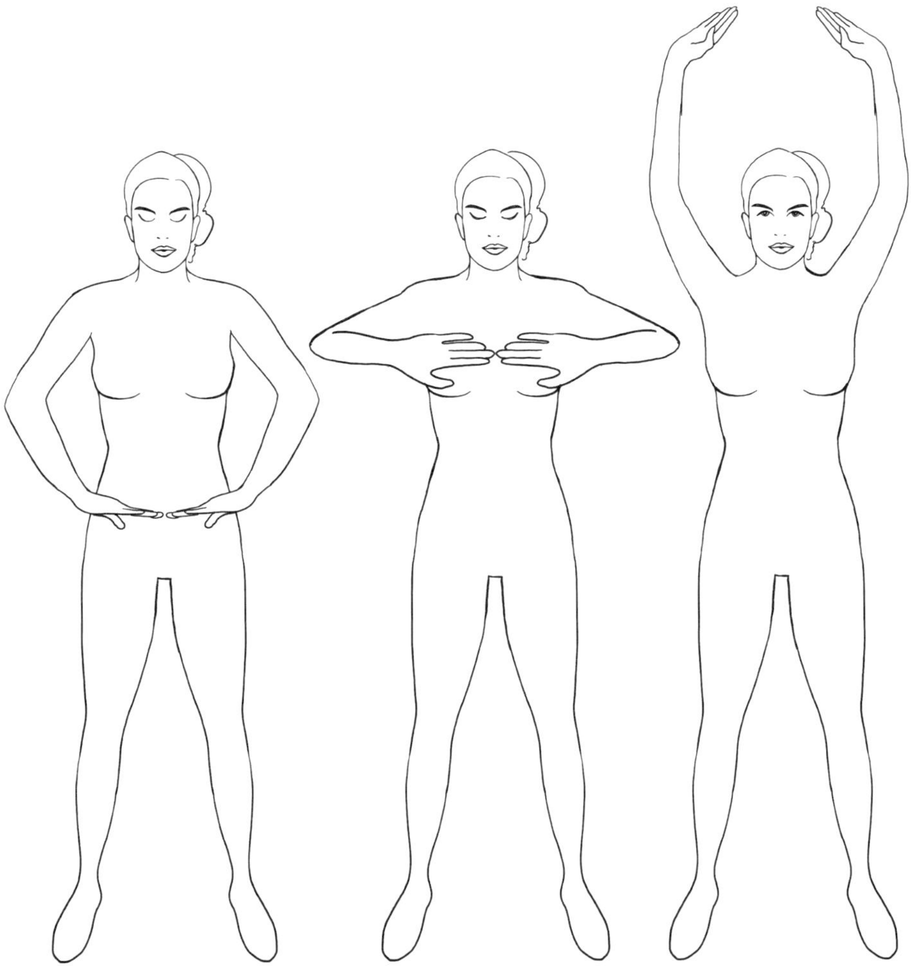

PART 2

YANG SHENG IN PRACTICE

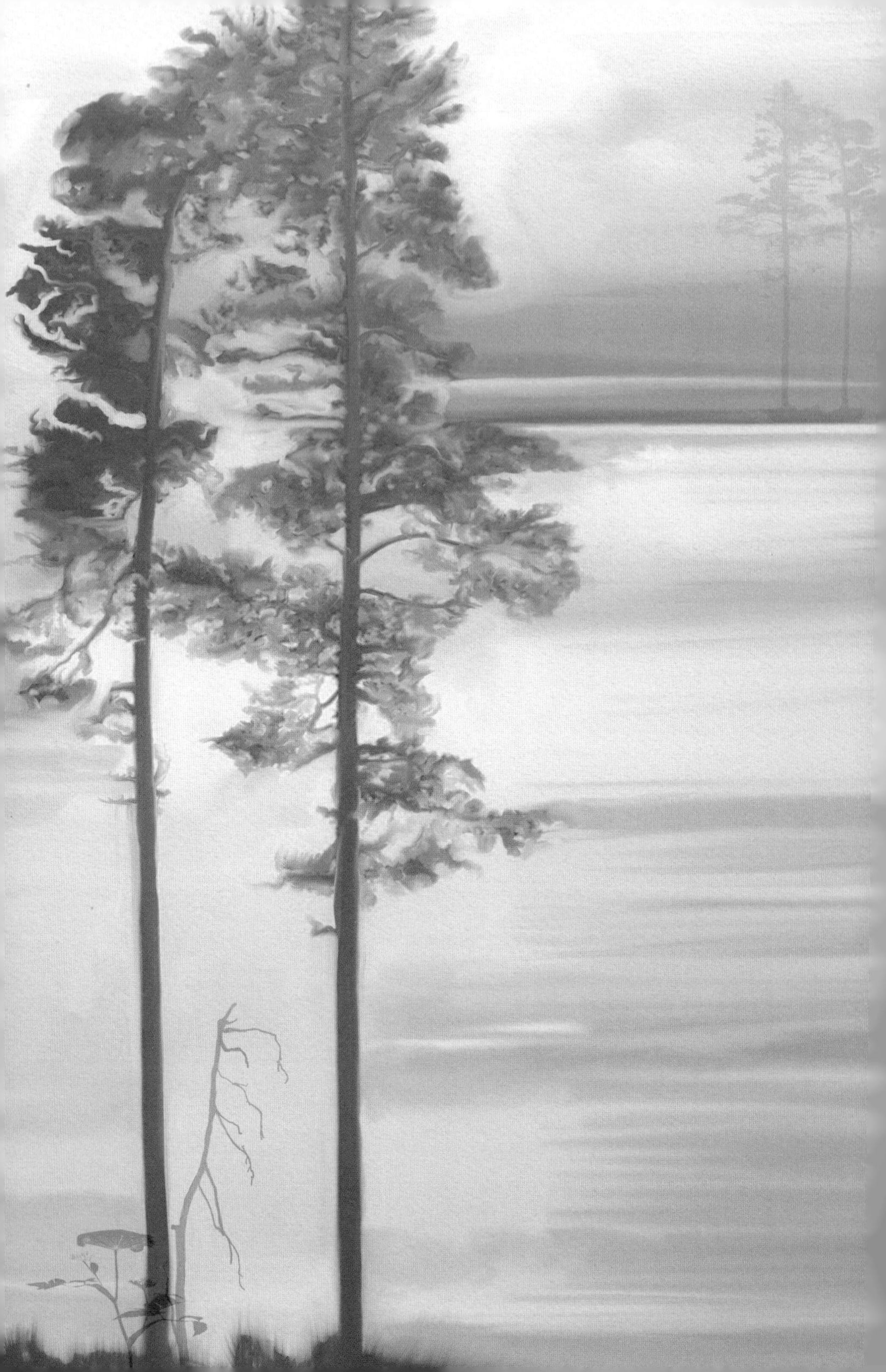

CHAPTER 1

BREATH

How to breathe better for calm, energy and stress release

'The perfected breathe all the way to their heels, unlike ordinary folk who only breathe as far as their throats.'

ZHUANGZI, 3RD CENTURY BCE

Breathing is something most of us don't pay much attention to. It just happens. But think about this: your very life started with an inhale. You could live for weeks without food and for days without water, but you could only survive minutes without breath. Breath is at once profound, subconscious and crucial to our very existence.

In Chinese medicine, breathing is thought of as the most vital function of all. You might think this is stating the obvious, but most of us haven't tapped into how effective using the breath to reach a state of relaxation can be. Breathing is the most immediate and powerful self-healing cure you have, a cornerstone of your health management. And it's one of only a few automatic bodily processes that you can control consciously.

That's why the One-Minute Rescue Breath Ritual (see page 38) is often one of the first things I teach in clinic.

The result is immediately clear: after three breaths, you can actually see and feel the person relaxing in front of you.

Right now, stop and pay attention to exactly how you are breathing. Have you just taken a deep breath because I mentioned it? Is this how you usually breathe? Or do you only breathe deeply during yoga or meditation?

For most of us, shallow breathing – and even stopping breathing for seconds at a time – has become our default, even more likely when we're stressed or busy. The Taoist approach is to make breathing deep into the abdomen your norm. The aim is to breathe evenly, but at a very slow pace, never holding your breath.

In Chinese medicine your diaphragm is said to hold on to emotional traumas. And moving it, with deep breathing or gentle exercise, helps release this. This idea should make sense: when we're with an upset person, we often tell them to take slow, deep breaths instead of short, sharp panicky ones.

The good news is, once you make breathing properly a habit, you'll feel calmer. In this section, you'll learn breathing exercises to do every day. Attach them to a regular activity – for me it's when I'm in the bath or shower – so they become a habit. I've also included some exercises for stressful situations and emergencies. During the day, try to breathe properly whenever you remember – and especially when you catch yourself breathing shallowly or holding your breath.

BREATHING AND STRESS

Chinese medicine has a poetic way of describing how deep breathing can bring you back out of your emotions into your rational, thinking mind: the heart is called the 'Emperor', while the lungs are called the 'Prime Minister'. So, taking deep breaths is asking your Emperor to listen to his Prime Minister and to listen to your rational mind.

The link between breathing and stress is becoming clearer. Studies have shown controlled, slow breathing stimulates the vagus nerve, which connects your head and stomach. This, in turn, prompts your parasympathetic nervous system – the rest and relax system – to kick in. The explanation in Chinese medicine is that slow, considered breathing takes you from an active, yang phase into a relaxed, passive, yin phase. This makes it the simplest form of meditation.

Lots of the other yang sheng techniques you'll be learning have been shown to have an effect on the vagus nerve, too. This is why it's worth doing these and any relaxation techniques regularly: practise appears to improve your vagal tone, meaning the more often you trigger your rest and relax phase, the easier it becomes.

BREATHING AND ENERGY

In Chinese wisdom, good breathing is one of two major ways (see page 28) to improve the quality of your qi (energy) and blood.

A Western explanation might be that to have energy, you need your blood to be oxygenated. In studies, controlled deep breathing has been shown both to increase oxygenation of the blood and improve circulation.

You might have tried various breathing exercises in yoga class or during meditation. Taoist breathing has similarities with yogic-type breathing: instructions often include slowing and lengthening the breath and combining particular positions with breathing. There are also fundamental differences, the main one being that in Taoist breathing you never hold or restrict the breath or block your nostrils.

THE CHINESE SMILING BREATHS

You may have already tried the One-Minute Rescue Breath Ritual (see page 38). I hope so; everybody can find the odd minute for this – on the school run, on hold to a call centre, even waiting for the kettle to boil!

I was taught this by John Munro of Long White Cloud Qigong, my fantastic qigong teacher, but many other masters also extol its virtues. On retreats you tend to practise this at dawn and dusk, as part of a full qigong session. I adapted the one-minute version from this full technique. You can start with just one breath, then if you like it, do five per more. If you enjoy those, keep going!

Breathe in as in the One-Minute Rescue Breath Ritual (see page 38). Then as you exhale, gently send an inner smile into each of your organs in turn – liver, kidneys, lungs, heart, stomach. For each organ, do three full rounds of breath, imagining it being filled with warmth and happiness.

Each organ is associated with a particular emotion; if you are feeling overwhelmed by one specific emotion, you can breathe into that particular organ only.

- To dissolve anger, smile into your liver.
- To dissolve fear, smile into your kidneys.
- To dissolve grief, smile into your lungs.
- To dissolve sadness, smile into your heart.
- To dissolve anxiety, smile into your stomach.

TWO EXERCISES FOR ENERGY

These two walking exercises come from the Chinese martial art of qigong. You may have seen people practising this slow series of movements in parks in the UK. In China, it's a morning ritual for millions.

There are lots of walking qigong exercises, but I've chosen two that are easy to do almost anywhere. Walking is the simplest way to integrate breath and movement and it's great because it doesn't require any extra time. Just the motion of walking stimulates qi, helping it flow better, and helps regulate yin and yang. The idea is consciously, to co-ordinate your breath with your steps, a type of meditation you may find easier than sitting.

If the exercises feel a little too much, you can get the benefits simply by focusing on your breath and being purposeful every time you walk. All these little pockets of focus throughout the day will add up.

QIGONG WALKING

Often called natural walking by qigong teachers, this isn't striding around with your thoughts all over the place. Instead, you focus on keeping your muscles relaxed and your breath regular. Ideally your walk should last 20 to 30 minutes but it's worth doing for shorter periods too, even for the 30 seconds between your desk and the kettle.

- Step out with your heel down and your toes up, keeping your neck straight and facing forward.
- Swing your arms naturally. Open the armpits so your arms are slightly out to the sides.
- Focus on stepping lightly and taking small steps. It may feel like you are using your heels more than normal; you'll get used to it.
- Keep your inhale and exhale the same length; for example, four counts in and four counts out. Focus on this and on the movement of your limbs. If your mind wanders, gently bring it back.
- Aim for 60 to 70 steps per minute. This is a fair pace, but it shouldn't leave you out of breath.

COUNTING STEPS

Breathe in for the time it takes you to do four steps. Breathe out for the time it takes to do eight steps. Aim to land on the floor with as little sound as possible. As you walk, keep your hands slightly raised, at the height of the hips, fingers facing forward and palms towards the ground. Imagine them sliding along a flat surface as you move. You can walk for as little or as long as you like.

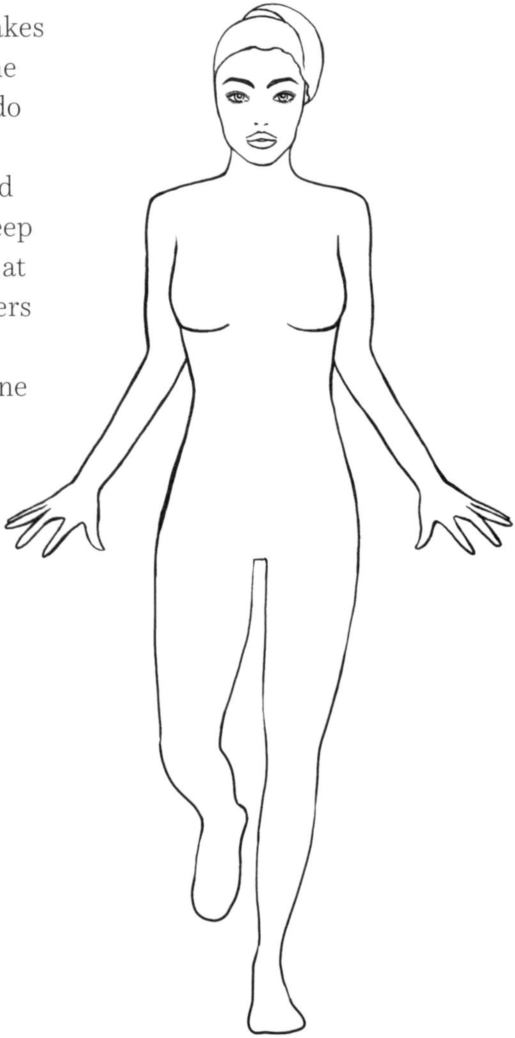

A NIGHT-TIME TUNE-UP

The six healing sounds

This is one of the oldest forms of breath therapy. It's becoming better known now, probably because it's so brilliant. The premise is that specific sounds correspond to the vibrations of each organ and its meridian. It feels and sounds strange, but I've experienced its transformative power firsthand.

If you can, do this daily, in particular before bed if you have trouble sleeping. In terms of noise level, you can tailor the volume to your environment. It's worth doing this in private if you find that making the sounds loudly gives you more of a release, but practising them really softly, almost under your breath, is better for long-term results.

Each organ you're working on is considered a 'master organ' in Chinese medicine, which means they control other organs and systems in the body. The idea is, if you keep your master organs happy and healthy, you'll stay in balance.

As you breathe a long breath out, make the sound. As you do so, visualise the matching organ or area. Send it happy vibes and imagine old, stale energy coming out of it, like mist. Repeat five times for each organ. Ideally, do three rounds.

1. Sssssss for your lungs.
2. Chooooo for your kidneys.
3. Shhhhhhhh for your liver.
4. Haaaaaaa for your heart and small intestine.

5 Whoooo for your stomach, spleen and pancreas.
6 Herrrrrrrr for your triple burner/san jiao (this roughly translates as your trunk or core).

A SIMPLE STRESS RELEASE

LAUGHTER QIGONG

Nothing beats laughing so hard you can't stop while tears stream from your eyes, right? We say laughter is the best medicine – and the ancient Chinese would agree. The theory is, the vibrations caused by laughter have an emotionally and physically healing effect on your body. You don't have to laugh in a specific way as the body can't tell the difference between laughter that just happens and the kind you force. Anyway, you'll find fake laughing quickly turns into genuine giggles. As laughing is so contagious, it's good to do this exercise with a friend. Google laughter qigong for some lovely, infectiously funny videos to get you started.

1 Stand with your feet hip width apart, bending your knees slightly.
2 Inhale, raising your arms to each side, wrists loose and palms facing towards the ground.
3 As you exhale, just laugh.

SIX PLANTS FOR AIR AND ENERGY

In the Chinese art of feng shui, plants are often used to activate positive qi in the home. As well as looking beautiful, plants have been shown to improve air quality by removing pollutants. A study from NASA named the best plants for purifying the air in your house or at work; the six I've included below are all used to attract energy in feng shui, too. As the name suggests, the money tree is said to attract money, so it's a good one to start with!

- Bonsai
- Snake plant*
- Chinese evergreen*
- Money tree*
- Chrysanthemum*
- Bamboo palm

*Toxic to animals and children if ingested.

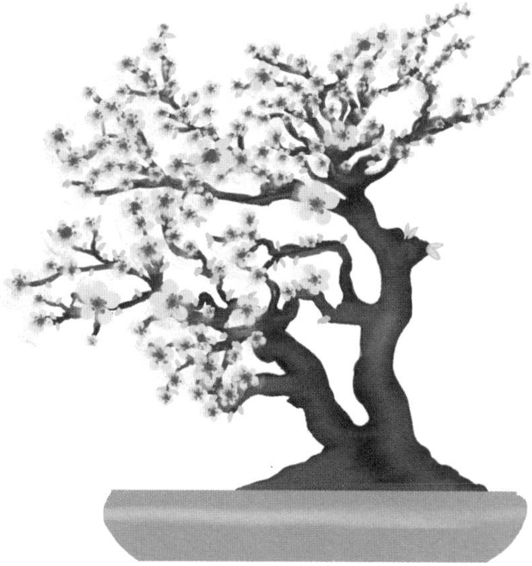

FIVE WAYS TO BREATHE BETTER

1 The air in your house might be more polluted than that outside. Research from the University of Surrey shows that inside air can become contaminated by everything from household cleaning materials to paints and fungal spores. Open the windows regularly to air the house or use an air purifier daily.
2 Sleep with your windows open. In one study, fresh air not only helped improve subjects' sleep quality, but they also reported noticeably less sleepiness and better concentration the next day, too.
3 If you've been travelling, as soon as you get close to some fresh air, especially around nature – a tree, a green space, the sea – take a few long, deep breaths.
4 Is your bra too tight? Over-tight underwired bras can restrict the movement of the ribs and diaphragm. Switch to a non-wired bra or yoga top, even if it's only while you're relaxing at home.
5 Download a gong app and set it to sound every hour while you're working. When it goes off, take a few deep, slow breaths. Remember, make your exhale longer than your inhale.

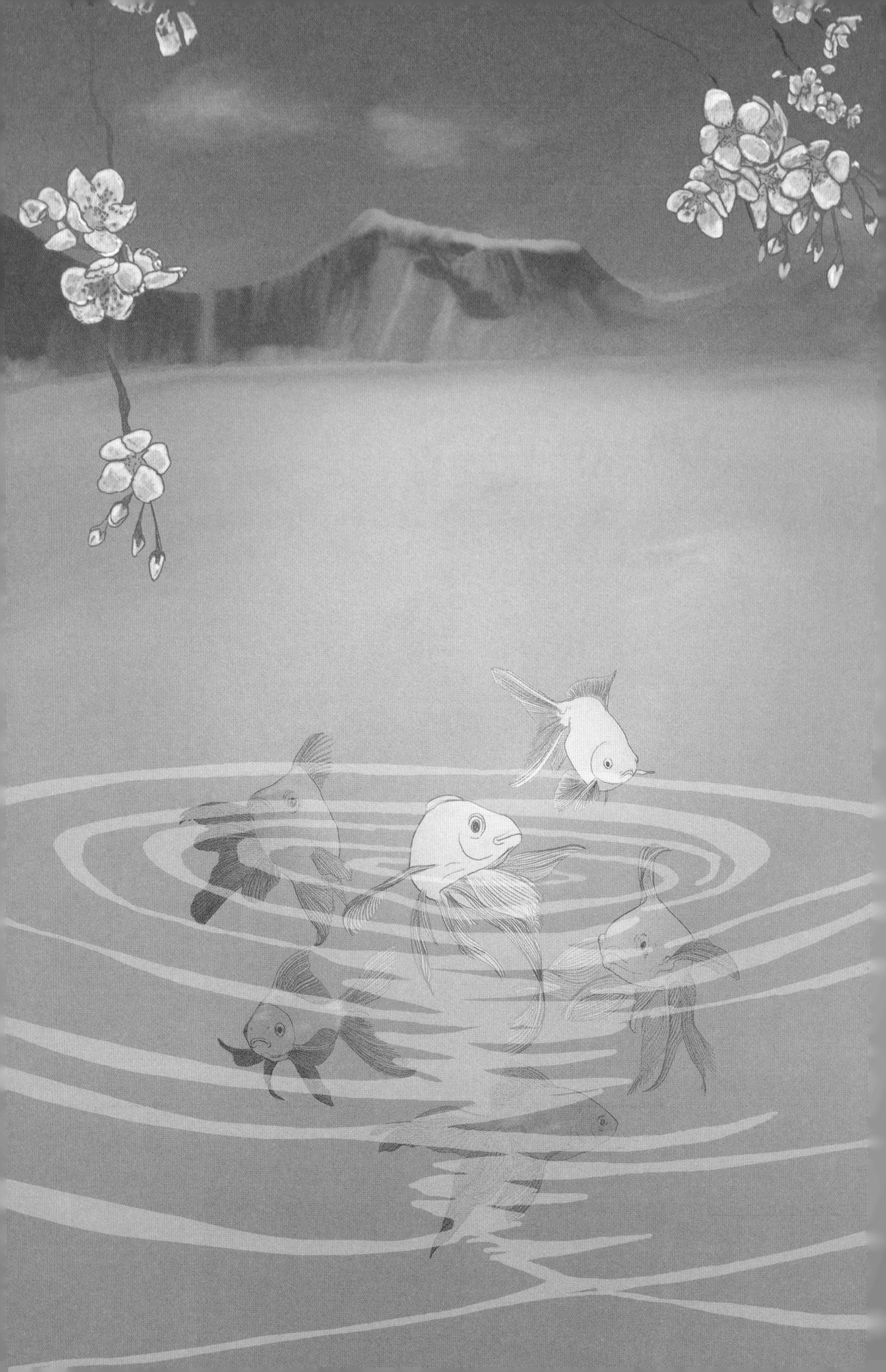

CHAPTER 2

DIGESTION

Changing how you eat to
transform how you feel

'He that takes medicine and neglects diet, wastes the skills of the physician.' CHINESE PROVERB

What really stands out about the Chinese attitude to food is the focus on digestion, on *how* you're eating. Whole schools of thought were developed as far back as the 12th century, stressing 'the importance of preserving stomach qi' for good health. For thousands of years, Chinese practitioners have been preaching that digestion and gut health are vital for both body and mind.

It's only been in the past ten years or so that Western medicine has come around to this way of thinking. Whereas the gut used to be considered simply a place for digestion and a small part of the immune system, it's now thought that a healthy microbiome – the millions of good bacteria that live in your gut – is the seat of good health.

There are now over 50,000 research papers on the microbiome and decoding the intricate interplay of how your gut affects both physical and mental health. Did you know the

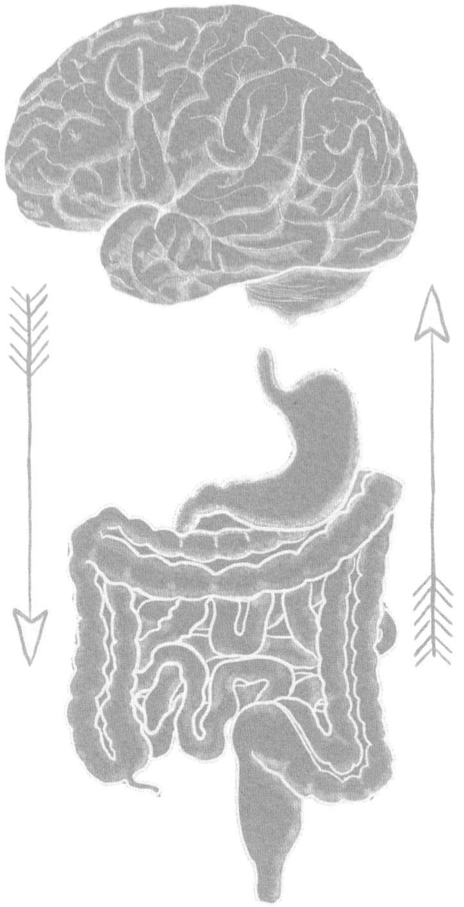

digestive system has its own nervous system, for example, with more nerve cells than the entire spinal cord? Or that over 90 per cent of the mood hormone serotonin is found in the gut?

You've likely felt the digestion-mind link in your own body: when you overeat, you feel sluggish in body and brain.

And when you feel nervous, you can often have 'butterflies' in your stomach or feel nauseous.

Chinese thinking about digestion ties your emotions very closely to the processing of food, too. The stomach is paired with the spleen in Chinese medicine, to make up the main organs of digestion. And interestingly, these organs also have the function of digesting sensations and information.

HOW TO DIGEST BETTER

In Chinese wisdom, stress is seen as bad for digestion, causing stagnation (blockages in your body's flow of qi). So, all these eating suggestions have one root: to give your digestion the time and space it needs to work properly as you live your full-on life. As well as these specific exercises, it's also a good idea, throughout the day, to recalibrate your body to its rest phase, as this is also its digest phase (see One-Minute Rescue Breath Ritual, page 38). Here are some simple steps to help you get the best from your food.

Love your food

In a Western understanding of the body, saliva begins digestion, making food easy to swallow and starting the breakdown of starches. But it has a bigger role according to Chinese medicine, where it's considered incredibly important for health. And it's said your emotions affect the quality both of your saliva and of your digestive juices. As

Taoist Master Mantak Chia has written, some Taoist texts refer to swallowing saliva up to 1,000 times a day for health. And Taoists say when you are relaxed, something called 'the longevity hormone' is released into the saliva.

If you mindlessly rush your food or, worse, feel guilty after eating, this is bad for the quality of your saliva. The same is true for eating while angry or bitter. If this sounds like you, it's fine to eat well 70 per cent of the time, and for the other 30 per cent to eat what you like – but do try not to attach guilt or any other negative emotions to food.

Before you eat

Zen master and spiritual leader Thich Nhat Hanh has some wise words on the subject of food and gratitude, very much in line with Taoist beliefs. He prescribes that while waiting for your food you should 'enjoy breathing for your nourishment and healing. Be grateful that you will soon have lovely food – and turn waiting into joy'. Be especially grateful if you're not having to cook! If you are cooking, give it your full focus and enjoy the process of creating for people you love (even if it's only for you).

Now sit down

The Chinese way is to sit down at a table to eat, rather than in front of a screen or at a desk. Eating in a calm atmosphere makes it easier for your body to be in rest and digest mode.

Look at your food

In China, food is usually displayed in the middle of the table to create a sense of abundance. And in Chinese medicine, the stomach meridian starts in the eyes. Looking before you eat encourages saliva production and tells your digestive system it's about to start work.

Chew, chew, chew

Well-chewed food – which in Chinese medicine means the food has turned into liquid and so has been mixed with air and qi – goes into the stomach ready for the next stage of digestion. Your stomach doesn't have teeth, so if you don't chew well, you're more likely to get indigestion or constipation.

Eat slowly

Your brain takes 20 minutes to recognise you're full, which is one reason eating with chopsticks is good. It reduces the size of a mouthful and slows down the eating process. Even when you're only having a sandwich, eat slowly.

Eat the same amount at each meal

Portion size is not a new idea. A Taoist scripture called *Nei-yeh,* thought to date from the 4th century, says: 'Overfilling yourself with food will impair your vital energy and cause your body to deteriorate. Over-restricting your consumption causes the bones to wither and the blood to congeal.'

You need to find the amount that's right for you. Ao Ying, a famous Chinese doctor, said that 'Man should endure 30 per cent hunger and 70 per cent fullness'. If stopping at 70 per cent full feels too different from your usual mode of eating, try stopping at 80 per cent to start with. Once you get the hang of it, you'll notice how much more comfortable your digestion feels.

Rest after eating

Instead of getting up from the table straight away, sit for 20 minutes after eating, to allow your digestion to get to work without interruption.

Don't drink during meals

Drinking any liquid with food not only stretches your stomach but also dilutes digestive juices. You can drink a small cup of tea before food to prepare the stomach and another around 20 minutes afterwards.

WHEN TO EAT

Energetically, Chinese medicine says the digestive system needs regularity, continuity and moderation. The prescription is to leave four- to five-hour gaps between meals to allow the digestive process time to work. Which ideally means no snacks, sorry.

Try to eat your meals when stomach qi, in charge of digestion, is at its strongest. Those times are: breakfast between 7am and 9am and lunch between 11am and 1pm. Dinner should be between 6pm and 7pm, to allow full digestion before bed.

If you follow this schedule, it will give you a natural fasting time between 7pm and 7am. Please note, this schedule absolutely does not mean you should starve yourself. It's about regulating the time between meals if you can, not getting over hungry – and especially not getting hangry!

Interestingly, Western research is now increasingly finding evidence that a longer overnight break from food may be helpful, allowing your gut microbiota time to work on spring-cleaning your gut. Overnight fasting may also have benefits for blood sugar control, metabolism, muscle mass, brain function and even mood.

THE GREEN TEA CEREMONY

'Better to be deprived of food for three days, than tea for one.'
Ancient Chinese proverb

When the Chinese talk about tea, they usually mean green tea. You might have tried it and not liked it. Maybe you found it bitter or didn't like the taste of the mouth-drying tannins? This could be because the tea was brewed from a low quality tea bag, or with boiling or too-hot water, which decreases the aroma, or was left to stew for too long.

You don't need to go to China to get good-quality tea, but do buy the best you can afford and give it the respect it deserves. When I serve my tea in clinic, people always say how delicious it is. It's the best drink, if done properly. Whether you're using loose leaf or tea bags, use water at 80°C/176°F, just off the boil. And steep for two to three minutes, no longer.

Aside from the buzz you get from the caffeine, green tea also contains an amino acid called L-Theanine. It has an anti-anxiety effect, which is what gives tea its calm plus energy effect. You've probably read about green tea's other impressive claims: it's thought to have cancer-fighting properties, be good for brain function, help control blood sugar and boost metabolism, help with fat digestion and even weight loss. Drink three to five cups a day, preferably in a nice tea cup – not a coffee mug!

HOW TO DRINK

Chinese medicine has no overall rules about what and how much to drink. Although it does say that, energetically, the best time to drink is in the middle of the afternoon. The general principle of avoiding excess applies to fluids too. Because we are all different, the advice is to use your thirst as a guide. Sugary drinks, including processed juices, aren't recommended, although vegetable juice does count as a vegetable. Oh, and avoiding excess applies to alcohol, too. That said, alcohol is used medicinally, to invigorate the circulation of blood. So, a glass or two won't derail your yang sheng journey, especially in winter.

HOT VS COLD

The whole modern obsession with salads being healthy and raw food being health food doesn't sit easily with Chinese medicine theory. It descibes the stomach as a bubbling cauldron, full of digestive fires that are put out by cold. So any raw food will sit, undigested, in your stomach. Ideally, don't eat food straight from the fridge, as both food and drink should be at room temperature. And you shouldn't really ice drinks.

THE FIVE TASTES: EAT FOR HEALTH

From a Chinese medicine perspective, the idea of going on a diet is absurd. Not only because diets are mentally stressful, but also because they deprive the body of nourishment and energy. Chinese medicine has no strict food exclusions – no 'raw only', 'carb-free' or 'high protein' rules. And, as you might have experienced, cutting out certain foods will only make you crave them more, before the inevitable rebound or binge, which is why most restrictive diets don't work in the long term.

For good health, variety is key. Or as the Chinese (and most likely your granny) would say, 'moderation in all things'. The idea is, balance in what you're eating gets your body into balance, then you'll no longer have cravings or need to overeat. Eventually, you will find your natural weight.

For a balanced plate, ideally include each of the five key tastes: sour, salty, bitter, spicy/pungent, sweet. This may seem strange, but think of appetite in terms of satisfaction – doesn't a meal feel most complete with a little of every flavour and not too much of a single one?

That said, what you might think of as being the flavour of a particular food or herb may not be the same as its Chinese taste classification. For example, broccoli is classified as 'bitter' and millet as 'salty'. The taste relates more to an intrinsic property of the food. You can find a table of the taste classifications and their foods on page 181.

WHAT IF YOU HAVE CRAVINGS?

Food cravings are seen as a sign of an imbalance in the body, as each of the tastes is linked to an organ, its function and its associated emotions. If you have a craving, have a little of the taste you crave – but in moderation. So, sweet potato is better than chocolate, a little chilli on the side rather than a mouth-blasting curry. Otherwise you risk causing another imbalance by creating new, rebound cravings.

- If you're changeable and erratic, eat a little more spicy food.
- If you feel nervous, eat a little more sweet food.
- If you're overweight, eat a little more sour food.
- If you feel sluggish, eat a little more bitter food.
- If you feel aggressive, eat a little more salty food.

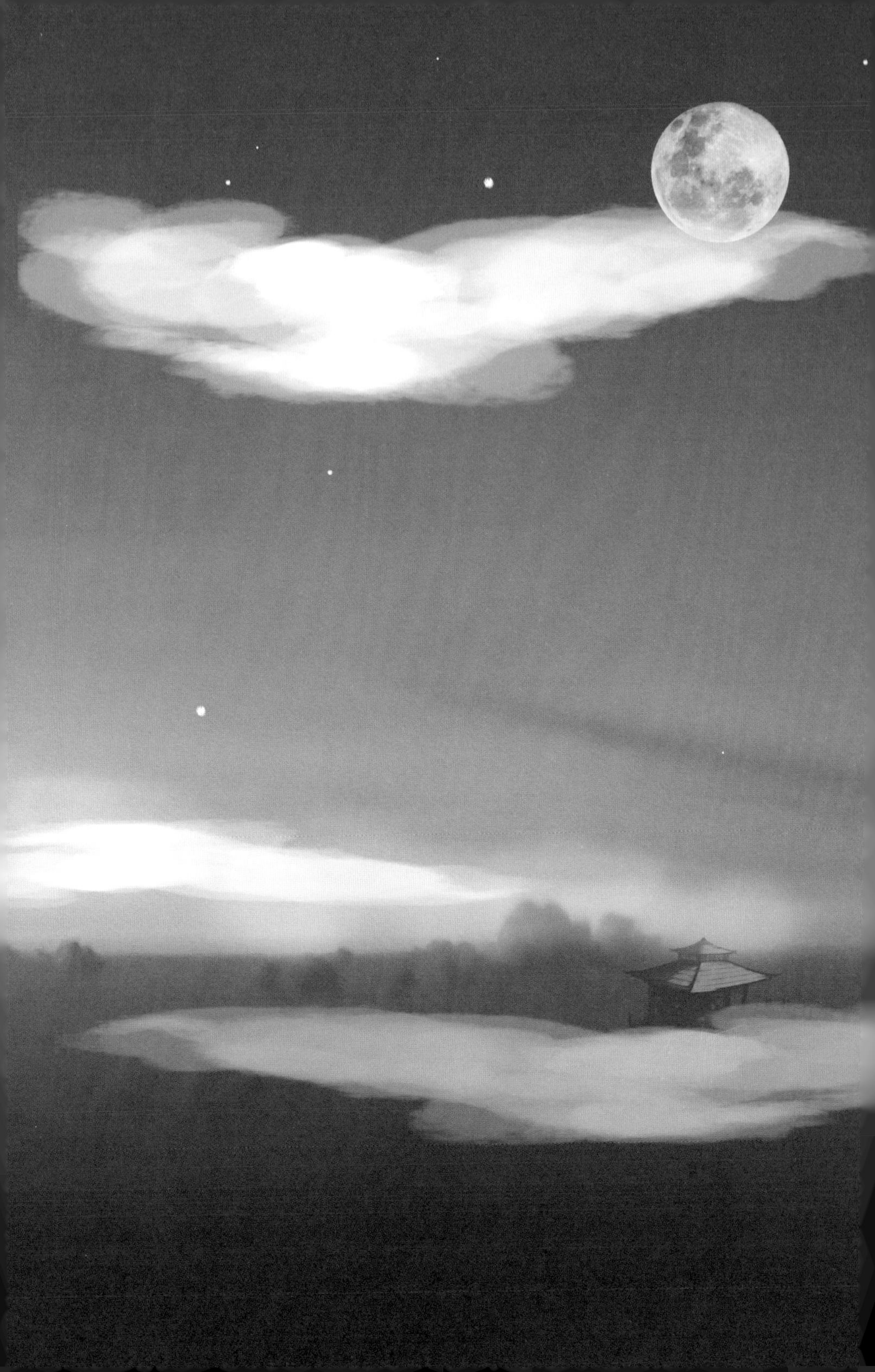

CHAPTER 3

SLEEP

What to do during the day to sleep well every night

'Sleep is the golden chain that ties health and our bodies together.' THOMAS DEKKER

After a night of fractured sleep, you know how terrible you feel. The silent fallout isn't great either: research shows even one night of sleep deprivation impairs your memory and affects your emotional state, hormones and appetite. And long-term insomnia is linked with a myriad of health problems.

Such is its importance, that asking after your sleep is one of the first questions you'll be asked during a Chinese medicine diagnosis. That's because sleep issues aren't just about sleep; they reveal numerous imbalances in your body.

In clinic, I find people usually fall into three groups: they can't get to sleep, they wake up in the early hours of the morning and can't get back to sleep. Or, if they're very unlucky, both. Some of them have tried sleeping pills. But, if so, they usually say they don't want to take pills and that medication leaves them tired in the morning.

Happily, as we're coming from a yang sheng approach, imbalances that lead to bad sleep can often be treated or prevented by lifestyle changes and simple exercises. If you feel you've tried everything but nothing's worked, yang sheng might have some of the answers.

That said, when it comes to sleep hygiene, Chinese medicine often does align with the expert advice you'll have heard before: keep your room quiet, cool and dark; have a gentle wind-down during the evening; and no screens right before bed. You probably know all this stuff already, but it's possible that you're not doing it! Try to think of your evenings as a transition from day to night, not a time to squeeze in more work. They are for gentle, not full-on, socialising, an opportunity to unwind.

HOW CHINESE MEDICINE LOOKS AT SLEEP

While the Chinese and Western advice might seem similar on the surface, the reasoning behind it is very different.

If you can't sleep, the first assumption in Chinese medicine would be that you have a yin/yang imbalance. Think of yang energy as a flame that keeps you warm, energised, powered up and motoring on all day. At night, yin energy should take over. It is cooling, nourishing, restoring and replenishing you physically and mentally as you sleep.

There's a protective energy in the body called wei qi, which flows on the exterior of your body during the day, when it's classified as yang. At night, this energy moves to the interior and so becomes yin. However, a sedentary lifestyle or stress will stop your wei qi flowing freely, disrupting the pendulum swinging from yang to yin. That will make you miss out on deep, regenerative sleep.

The second assumption would be that your insomnia is signposting what's called an organ imbalance. Don't forget, Chinese wisdom views our organs in a more expansive way than Western biology, so this doesn't mean a medical issue. For example, if you need the loo frequently at night, Chinese medicine would say this points to a kidney imbalance, but this isn't the same as diagnosing a kidney infection.

The time of night you struggle to either get to sleep or wake up will point to which organ has the imbalance. Can you tie your sleep difficulty to a certain point in the night? Issues between 9pm and 11pm are connected to the functioning of the heart, 11pm to 1am is the gallbladder, 1am to 3am is the liver, 3am to 5am is the lung, 5am to 7am is the large intestine.

This probably sounds very unfamiliar, but the good news is, there are plenty of self-healing techniques for sleep in Chinese medicine.

TIMINGS FOR THE BEST NIGHT'S SLEEP

This is what not to do for good sleep: spend the evening on the sofa watching Netflix, scrolling Instagram and WhatsApp, then fall into bed at 11.30pm. Instead, take nature as your cue and try to transition slowly from day to night. Both East and West agree that establishing a consistent bedtime and sticking to it does improve sleep quality.

- **From 6pm to 7pm:** Eat your main meal. The ancient Chinese observed that going to bed on a full stomach is bad for sleep, because digestion involves the warming and transformation of your food, which are very yang activities. Caffeine, spicy food and alcohol are considered yang, too, so are to be avoided if you can.
- **9pm:** Start your bedtime routine. Turn off the TV. Either soak in the bath or bathe your feet. Do some gua sha (see page 83). Tapping slowly and gently (see page 40) is also relaxing now, especially after your bath. Do it for 10 minutes – I wholly recommend a bamboo tapper. And have a look at the suggested evening routine on page 159.
- **10pm:** Aim to get into bed, leaving your mobile outside the room or turning it off. It's really important to get off screens and relax the eyes; the eyes are linked to the liver in Chinese medicine, and an overloaded liver will keep you awake. Turn off the power sockets at the wall, too; some people are sensitive to yang energy from mobiles, wifi and sockets. I'm often asked about bedtime supplements; I recommend Valerian tincture and also taking magnesium.
- **10.15pm to 10.30pm:** Turn off the light. Aim to be asleep by around 10.30pm. We enter our highest-quality state of sleep about 40 minutes after we fall asleep. And the hours between 11pm and 1am are when your liver repairs itself in Chinese medicine. If you don't get this early sleep, you'll wake less refreshed.

TECHNIQUES FOR THE BEST NIGHT'S SLEEP

Take yin breaks

Night is when your yin energy should naturally take over, allowing you to rest. But as we all lead such fast-paced and so very yang lives, it's easy to get out of the habit of winding down to allow this to happen. Yin and yang can get out of balance for many reasons, but stress is one of the biggest offenders. Do one or more of these techniques, and you'll find it easier to chill out later.

1 Lie down for a short rest or nap during the day to nourish your yin. As we naturally feel sleepy after lunch, this is the best time for an up-to-30-minute nap. If this isn't possible, 3pm to 5pm is also good. Even five minutes in a quiet spot, practising deep breathing, will help.
2 From 6pm, limit high-intensity exercise, such as running, gym, boxing – basically anything that revs you up and adds stress to your body. Take gentle exercise instead, outside if possible. Yoga, walking or swimming are all good.
3 Activate the rest phase of your nervous system repeatedly throughout the day, using the One-Minute Rescue Breath Ritual and the Chinese Smiling Breath techniques (see pages 38 and 52).

MINERAL BATH RITUAL

In the bath houses of China, treatment has a specific routine. I have shortened it here, so you can do it at home, but it's still hugely beneficial to induce a peaceful sleep. Always bathe first, gua sha afterwards. You can use any good quality, magnesium rich mineral salt, such as Epsom salts.

1. Hot water

Soak for 20 minutes in a bath that's as hot as you can manage. I don't advise immediate immersion into hot water. Instead, get into a bath of warm water, about a third full, then increase the temperature slowly. As you warm up, the relaxation response kicks in, your blood pressure decreases and your heart rate goes down.

2. Exfoliation

Exfoliate all over your body using a loofah or body brush, making sure you include your groin and armpit regions. Exfoliation is part of the traditional spa rituals of many cultures; historically, the Chinese used dried fruit and vegetable fibres fashioned into sponges. Exfoliation encourages lymphatic drainage and boosts immunity and circulation as well as leaving the skin super soft.

3. Cold water

Follow this with a cold shower, as cold as you can manage, for as long as you can manage. A regular blast of cold water – even 30 seconds – may help boost your immunity as well as your circulation and metabolism. In one study, for example, it reduced the severity of cold symptoms (although not the length of a cold). Next, turn the water to warm. Always end on warm at bedtime to relax you, but if you're doing this in the morning, end on cold for energy.

GUA SHA

Studies have shown gua sha switches you into relaxation mode, which is exactly where you want to be pre-sleep. Gua sha is especially helpful if you're chronically stressed and find it hard to make that switch automatically.

At bedtime, it's good to gua sha the chest and arms. Gua sha is calming and anti-anxiety because it helps to stimulate the flow of blood and qi around your heart and lungs. Press-stroke your chest from the centre outwards using a gua sha tool or metal teaspoon. Do six to eight times on each side. Next, do the same along your arms, working outwards.

Nightly quick and simple foot gua sha

Both foot baths and foot rubs are great sleep inducers, descending racing thoughts out of your monkey mind down into your feet, grounding you. Use a metal gua sha tool or a teaspoon to draw a figure of eight repeatedly on your sole, for a minute on each foot. Or slap each foot lightly with your cupped hand, 50 to 100 times on each foot.

The full pre-bed foot relaxation

Fill a bowl with warm water, adding magnesium salts for extra relaxation. Soak your feet for up to 20 minutes. If you break a sweat that's good, as it shows you are unblocking the meridians. But don't stay hot; excessive sweating uses up too much energy.

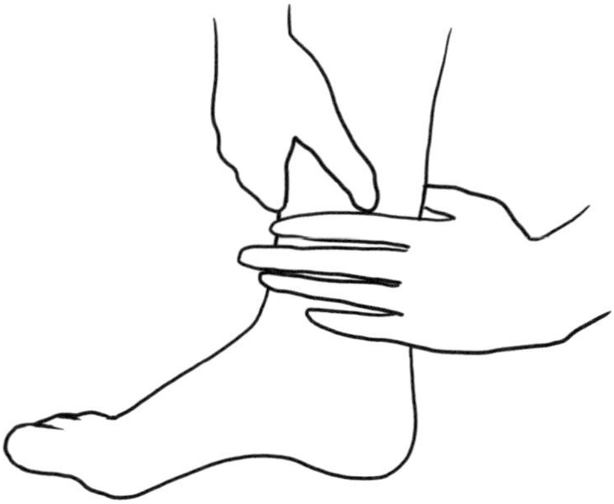

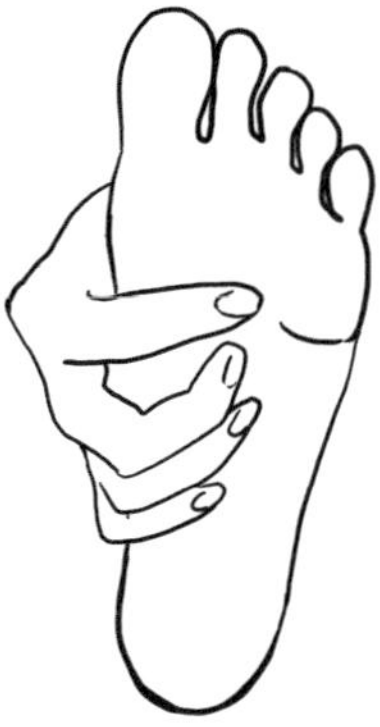

Now, activate an acupressure point called Spleen 6, good for nourishing yin. To locate it, place your hand over your inner leg at the bottom of your ankle. Spleen 6 is four fingers width up. Press and hold there for a few moments on each leg. Next, press and hold the sole of your foot, at a point that's widely used for insomnia, Kidney 1 (see diagram opposite).

THE SIX HEALING SOUNDS

Practising the six healing sounds – in particular the most relevant sound to the organ of your waking time (see page 79) – will get your body back into balance quickly. It will work no matter what the underlying issue, so is ideal if you are struggling to diagnose this. (See page 56 for the Six Healing Sounds.)

THE LIFTING THE SKY STRETCH

This ancient qigong stretch is a great all-round exercise. As well as balancing your energies before bed, you can do it to centre yourself any time you are feeling a bit out of whack. Learn it on page 42.

CAN'T SLEEP? SOS TREATMENTS

- Make a cup of chrysanthemum tea. It's said to clear excess yang energy and is really soothing for those times when your nerves are frayed.
- There's a useful acupressure point called Anmian, which translates as 'peaceful sleep'. It's a very slight dent around 2 cm behind the middle of your ear on the neck. Apply pressure with your finger and massage in a circular motion. The traditional instruction is to do this 100 times.
- Breathe to your feet. Take a deep breath in, feeling the air fill your stomach and imagining it continuing all the way down through your body to your feet. Chinese wisdom holds that qi follows intention. Intending the breath to move right down to your toes also focuses your mind and takes you out of your head and racing thoughts.

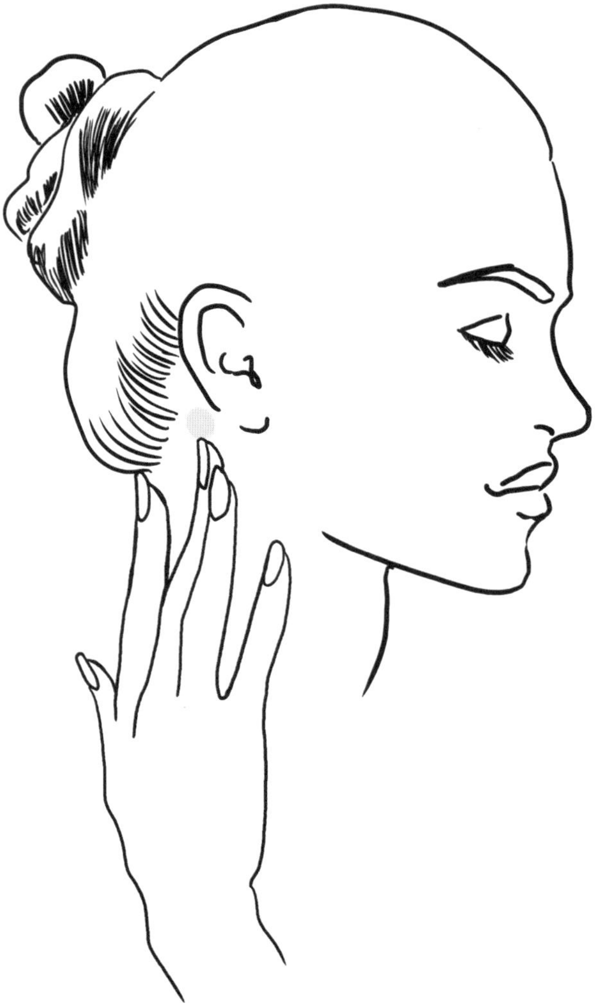

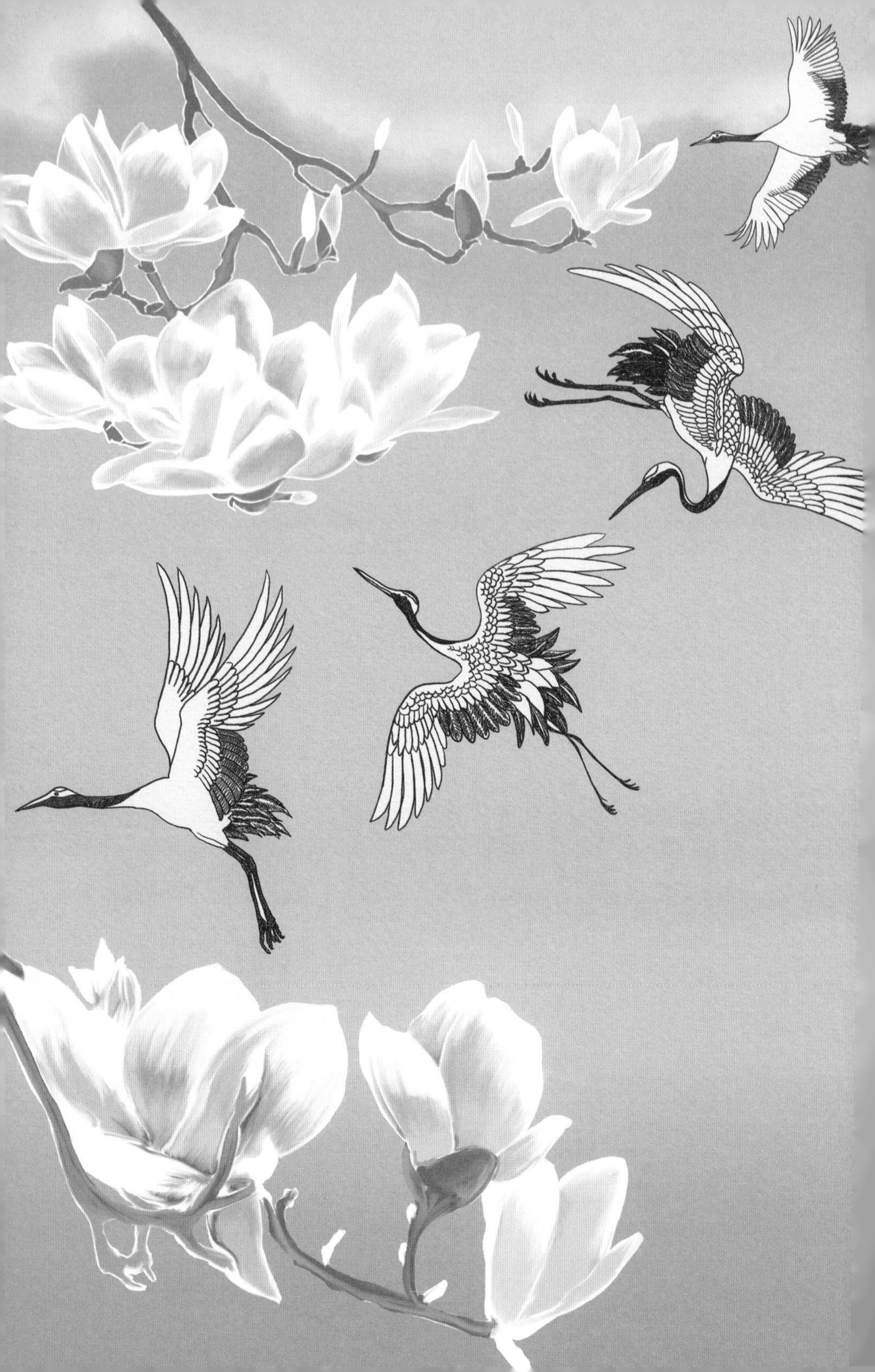

CHAPTER 4

EXERCISE

The best types of movement for health, strength and energy

'The hinges of a moving door never rust, and flowing water never stagnates.'
PHILOSOPHER AND LONGEVITY SPECIALIST
GE HONG, CE 300.

Have you ever started a fitness plan, maybe promised yourself you'll run or swim or gym every day? Then a week, a month or even a few days later, despite your very best intentions . . . it's over. You're off the workout wagon. Maybe you had a bad day at work and, understandably, took refuge in a bottle of wine instead of yoga. Or perhaps when the alarm went off, you were just too tired to drag yourself out of bed for a run.

The trouble with making a big, revolutionary exercise promise or plan is that it's all or nothing. So, the moment you don't reach 100 per cent, you end up doing nothing.

Or perhaps this is you: you exercise regularly, but you still feel tired most of the time. You've plateaued; you never seem to get much fitter or stronger or closer to the shape you want. You're demoralised. And every time you exercise, it's a huge effort to get started.

If so, exercising according to yang sheng principles will be a revelation. I can relate to all of the above and one of the most life-changing things I learnt from Chinese medicine is that exercise does not need to be strenuous, an effort to fit into your life, or indeed lengthy, to be effective.

Chinese wisdom has showed me that slogging it out in the gym or signing up for a marathon is not necessarily the best thing for my body – or yours. That is, unless you truly, deeply love doing these things, in which case, fine. In fact, in Chinese thinking, pushing yourself to do a super-strenuous workout, especially when you'd be better off resting or sleeping, is not only unsustainable but it's adding even more stress to your body, too.

THE MIRACLE OF INTERNAL EXERCISE

The kind of exercise I can promise will give you the body you want, a body that feels fit, strong and energetic, is internal exercise or meditative movement. This is any combination of slow, considered movements with breath and mental engagement, so it includes yoga, of course, and tai chi. But the emperor of internal exercise, the one that changed my body and is a fundamental pillar of Chinese medicine, is qigong.

Qigong is, quite simply, the ultimate self-healing technique, a way you can learn to manipulate qi around the body. Remember, for good health we are always looking for our qi to flow as freely as possible and qigong achieves this. It was invented as 'dynamic meditation', to allow Taoist masters to keep their muscles relaxed, supple and strong after hours of sitting meditation but without breaking their focus. Its roots can be traced back to the 8th century BCE, i.e. 10,000 years ago. By the 3rd century BCE, this practice had crystallised into the beginnings of qigong as it is today. You could say, qigong is so good people have been doing it for at least 5,000 years. There's nothing gimmicky or unproven about that!

If you've done a martial art or tai chi, the wide stance and relaxed, flowing movements of qigong will be familiar. Qigong forms the basis of all martial arts, so before trainees learn how to fight, they will always study it. Visit a Chinese community anywhere in the world and in public parks you'll see locals moving as one, doing this languid dance.

WHAT'S SO GOOD ABOUT QIGONG?

Previously, how you exercise may have been motivated by your looks. But it's when you realise you *feel* truly different that qigong will become a non-negotiable part of your life.

I would argue that just a few minutes a day can actually be more effective than a lengthy, strenuous workout, as long as you are moving in your day-to-day life. Or, if you're happy with your daily workout, you'll feel the benefits from adding just a few minutes of qigong.

So, why is it so good? In Chinese medicine, qigong is used for three main purposes: as a healing tool, as training for a martial art and to elevate the spirit. In modern terms, it's been shown to leave you feeling rejuvenated and more energetic, be deeply relaxing, to lower the heart rate and blood pressure and relieve pain, and may support the immune system, too.

You may be used to thinking about exercise as improving the way you look, or perhaps improving the health of your heart and lungs, but Chinese medicine says that while aerobic exercise does work those organs, it simultaneously taxes them. Qigong, on the other hand, works the muscles and nourishes all of the organs – but, crucially, doesn't strain them. It boosts your oxygen uptake and circulation, but while your body is relaxed. This builds your capacity to store and generate your reserves of qi.

Remember, according to Chinese medicine, your organs control the entire health of your body. This includes, amongst other things, your muscles, fascia, bones, body fat and any tendency towards weight imbalance. Look after your organs and you'll see a knock-on positive effect on all of your health. Qigong will give you stamina without stress, tone without pain. As you do the exercises, you're balancing the whole body and, because they're so gentle, they even suit older people and those who are recovering from illness. (If you're concerned, ask your GP before you undertake any exercise.)

TAI CHI OR QIGONG? WHAT'S THE DIFFERENCE?

To sum it up, if qigong is the grandmother, kung fu is the parent and tai chi is the child. Tai chi is a stylised martial arts form of qigong, rumoured to have been created by a Taoist master called Zhang Sanfeng in the 14th century. The story goes that he saw a magpie and a snake fighting in the forest and was inspired by the contradictory yet balanced nature of their battle.

To a beginner, the similarities between the two will stand out more than the differences. Both tai chi and qigong focus on using breath, body movement and visualisation to move qi around the body. But while each tai chi move can theoretically be used for self-defence, most qigong motions exist solely for the purpose of meditation, health and healing. And while tai chi is typically a highly choreographed and complex series of movements, qigong is easier to learn, a more repetitive practice that you can easily do at home. This makes it ideal as an effective self-treatment.

There are a lot of studies that show tai chi and qigong are incredible for health; the two are often used interchangeably in research. They have been shown to have a positive effect on muscle strength, flexibility and balance, to improve fitness and the endurance levels of the heart and lungs. One 2013 study concluded that tai chi was nearly as effective as jogging at lowering the risk of death! The Chinese government have recently adopted tai chi as a solution to help cut stress in the workplace.

BALANCE YIN AND YANG

You may be thinking: but can a few minutes of slow movement every day really replace a gym session? In fact, qigong can be a good cardio workout. It's one of the many things I love about it, that you can go as hard or as gently as you want. Have a play with the exercises: Swimming Dragon is a great one to start with. Try varying the intensity by speeding it up to raise your heart rate and slowing it right down for more stretch-based results.

If you want to stick with your usual gym session or hard run, you can get the fantastic benefits of qigong by doing any of the exercises in this chapter at the start and the end of your workout. This is stealing a really great trick from kung fu, called 'transitioning' the body.

There's good reason to do this, according to Chinese medicine: any exercise you do should both restore your nourishing yin energy and move your invigorating yang energy. A hard workout is very yang and stresses the body – and when your body is stressed, you'll never reach peak condition. However, by bookmarking your workout with qigong, you will increase yin energy, switch off stress and re-engage your rest phase, allowing your body to recuperate. Even if you don't have a lot of time, you're better off doing a shorter workout and slotting in a transition before and after.

YANG SHENG TECHNIQUES FOR HAPPY EXERCISE

Move your body first thing

Chinese wisdom advises that your yang qi – your active energy – rises in the morning, so just after sunrise is the best time of the day to move.

Punctuate your day with movement

Rather than tagging exercise onto your day, aim to do each of the seven daily qigong power exercises spread out over the day. Short bursts of moderate exercise have been shown to be as effective as one long workout. Try to reach 10,000 steps throughout the day, too. As I've said, too much exercise is not good for you, but neither is too little.

Do what you love

Choose something you love to do. If it's a pleasure, you'll make the time to do it and it'll become a regular part of your life. Whether it's kickboxing, Pilates, rock climbing, Zumba or just walking the dog, the right exercise can be one of the great joys of life. It gets you out of your head, helps you breathe better and sleep better. The Chinese explanation is that the heart, as well as pumping blood around the body, is also responsible for joy. If you approach your workout positively, you'll get this energetic benefit as well as the physical one.

Plan what you do

Goal setting has been a part of Chinese wisdom for millennia. Master Mantak Chia has a lovely way to describe goals: 'dreams with deadlines'. Once you've found what you enjoy doing, set a goal and a realistic plan to achieve it. It's really important to write down your goals – get them on paper and you'll become accountable.

Be consistent

You'll need a little discipline to make your goals happen. And even with exercise you love, discipline isn't always easy. So, start small, even if it's, 'I'll do one qigong exercise daily for a week'. You can begin with just one minute, as long as you are consistent. For practise to be effective, you need to do it every day. Over time, build up from that minute.

Look after your willpower

Chinese wisdom explains why your willpower deserts you when you are stressed or overtired or burnt out. The organ responsible for willpower is your kidneys – and this is also the first organ to be thrashed by the stress response. So when you are stressed, your kidneys need TLC, not to be hammered even more by exercise. If you feel burnt out, you need to slowly build up your kidney reserves. As above, start with just one minute of exercise and increase gradually. As humans, our willpower is naturally limited; it's best to get tiny habits ingrained before you progress to big ones.

Listen to your body

The Chinese sages rather starkly warn that 'stagnation is death', and it's true, you need to move. But if your days are spent stuck in an office and you feel exhausted by 5pm, dragging yourself to the gym after work isn't going to be good for either your body or your soul. If you're feeling tired or unwell, you don't have to exercise. You might be better to simply rest, if that's what your body is telling you. Or try a short meditation, such as the One-Minute Rescue Breath Ritual (see page 38) then a simple qigong exercise, such as Lifting the Sky (see page 42) to boost your energy.

SEVEN DAILY QIGONG POWER EXERCISES

These are the fundamental basics of your new exercise routine. I'm being this definite because I know doing these every day will make you feel energetic, strong, invigorated and positive. Add them to your regular workout, or on busy days they can be your only exercise. These five are in addition to Lifting the Sky (see page 42) and the One-Minute Tapping Ritual (see page 40).

Not sure you can fit them in? Think of it like having a shower. Even if you are travelling and crazy busy, you still have time to do that, right? The more you do these exercises, the quicker you'll see results but, most of all, consistency is key. Aim for one minute of each to start with. As always, start gently and build up slowly.

SHAKING

This really is as simple as it sounds, it's just shaking – all over, from top to bottom – which invigorates your entire circulatory system.

1 Start slowly and gently with your arms, then move on to your hands, your arms, your feet, your legs, your head, your trunk.

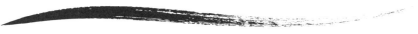

2 As you begin to feel your body relaxing and your qi flowing, build up the motion. If you are older, weak or unwell, go for more of a gentle, slow, swaying or rocking action.
3 Continue for a minute. But if it feels good, carry on for as long as you like.

TURNING THE WAIST

The exercise is great for releasing and relaxing your joints and encouraging your circulation.

1 Stand with your hips and feet facing forwards.
2 As you twist at the waist, swing your arms. Your hands should swing around and firmly pat your lower abdomen and back.
3 Do 30 seconds, then switch it up so that your hands come up as you twist and hit the back of your shoulders.

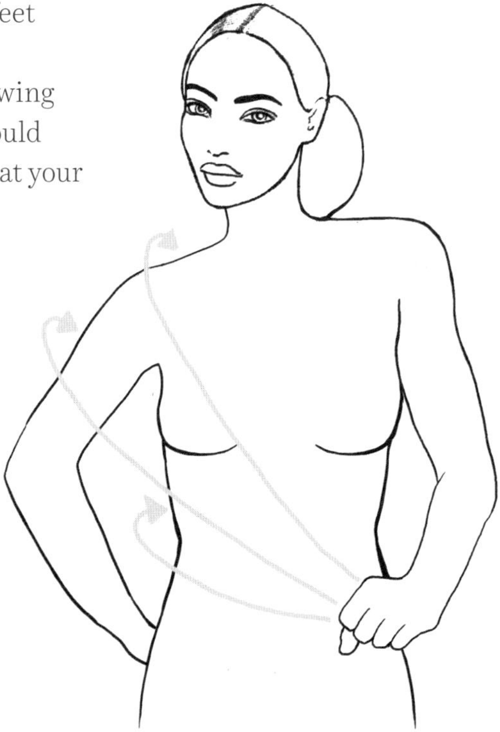

TIP TOES

This exercise improves your posture and encourages good digestion and balance, as well as toning your pelvic floor and strengthening your kidney energy.

1 Stand up straight, with your feet slightly wider than shoulder width apart.
2 Bend the knees.
3 Stretch your arms out in front of you, keeping your palms facing downwards.
4 Gently rise up high onto the balls of your feet. You'll need to shift your weight slightly forward to compensate and bend the knees.
5 Hold it for a second, then straighten your legs. Finally, put your heels down, back to the original stance.
6 Do this for at least one minute each day.

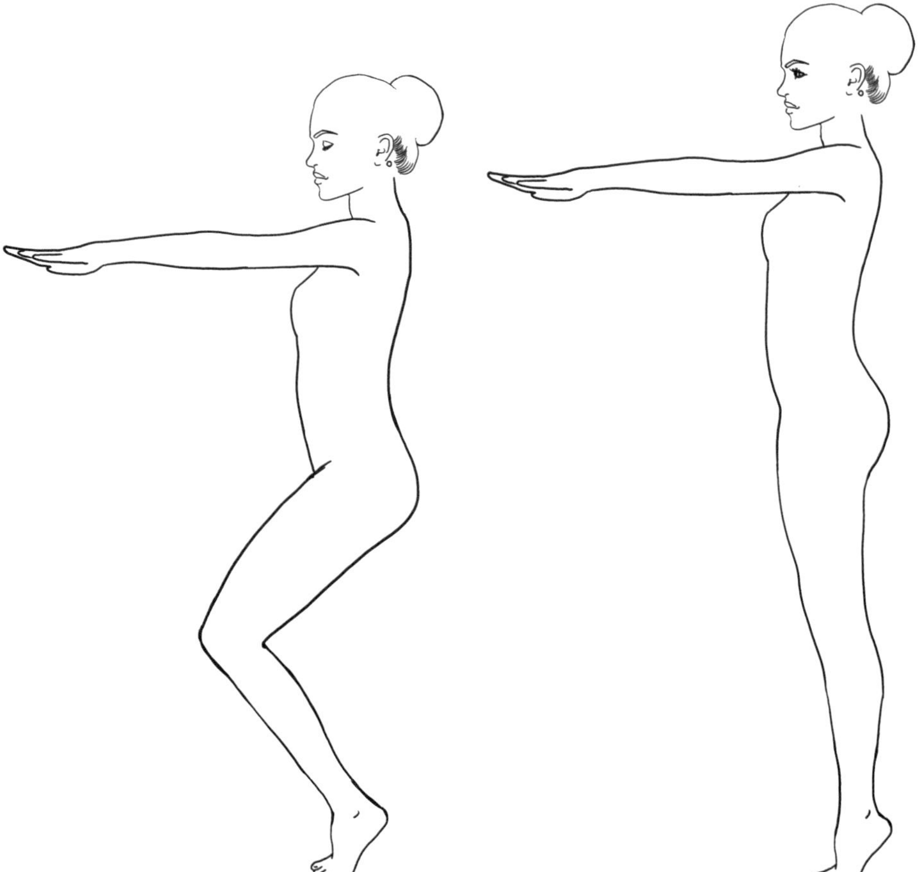

SWIMMING DRAGON

This all-encompassing movement helps to shape and firm the abdomen, improve overall balance and co-ordination and is used to support the kidneys and bones in Chinese medicine. As with all of these exercises, there's no need to push your body to its limit. If you have injuries or are feeling fragile, go slowly and pay attention to what feels good.

1 Stand with your feet together. Rub your hands together and place them in prayer position in front of your heart.
2 Engage your abdomen. Push your hip out to the left and take your hands, fingertips leading, still in prayer position, in the opposite direction, so your right arm is vertical. Keep your hands pressed together, to create a right angle between your hands and your wrist.
3 Swim your hands from one side to the other in a figure-of-eight loop, each time with your hips going in the opposite direction.
4 Keeping going, slowly swim your figure of eight down towards the floor, so you are doing it over your hips, then your knees.
5 Swim your way back up until your arms are now above your head.
6 Stretch your fingertips up, lifting up on your tiptoes as you do so.
7 Finally, bring your arms down and finish by resting your splayed hands on your belly, thumbs and digit fingers touching to make a heart shape. Repeat for one minute.

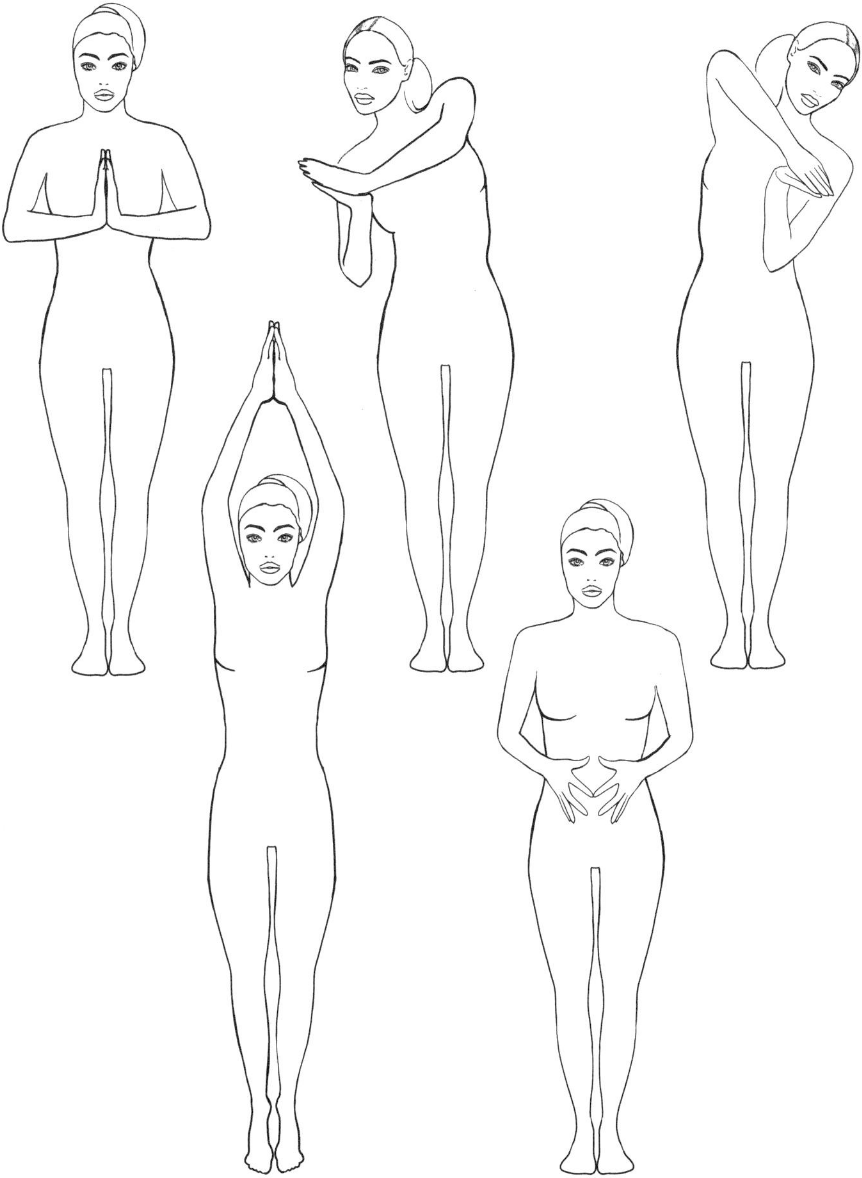

SPINNING MANDARINS

This exercise is also great for your abs, but is more aerobic than Swimming dragon.

1. Start with your feet wide apart.
2. Put a small object – a piece of fruit such as a mandarin or lemon is perfect – in each hand. Keep your hands flat. (The Chinese would traditionally hold saucers to perform this exercise, but fruit is less smash-able!)
3. Squat down, then stretch your right arm out diagonally in front of you, pushing out your hand as though you were offering the mandarin to someone just out of your reach.
4. Move the mandarin horizontally in front of you, up out over and behind your head, then bring it back in front into your centre, transferring your weight to follow the motion.
5. Repeat on the other side.
6. Do at least five reps on each side. This should take between one and two minutes.

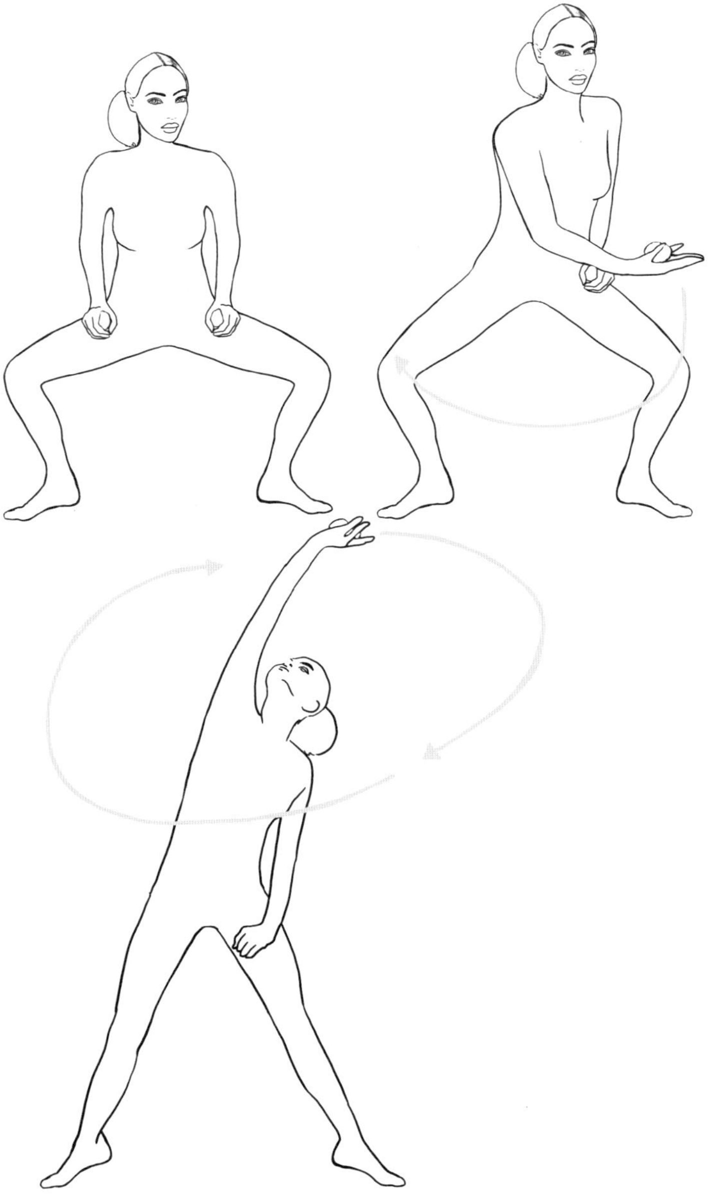

CIRCLE WALKING

This exercise helps your qi to flow smoothly in your body and is a great way to slot in a short burst of activity. It's particularly good after lunch or dinner, to help with digestion. There's an old Chinese folk saying: 'If you take 100 steps after each meal, you'll live to 99'. For the first five minutes (or half the time you want to do), walk to the right. Then change direction and walk to the left. Your circle can be as big or small as you like, from a few metres to the size of your local park.

SUPERCHARGE YOUR EXERCISE

Qigong should be performed outside if at all possible, to honour nature. In fact, it's better to do any exercise outdoors. Walking in a green space – taking deep lungfuls of fresh air, hearing the birds singing, having a sense of the weather changing, feeling cycles of growth and retreat – is, Chinese medicine says, nurturing to your soul. You inhale the qi of the natural world surrounding you, as well as absorbing it through your skin. If you can't get outside, the next best option is to make sure the room you're exercising in is well-ventilated – throw open the windows! – and, if possible, filled with plants. In addition, qigong teachers tell you to face east in the morning, north in the middle of the day, and south in the evening if you can, to take in more qi.

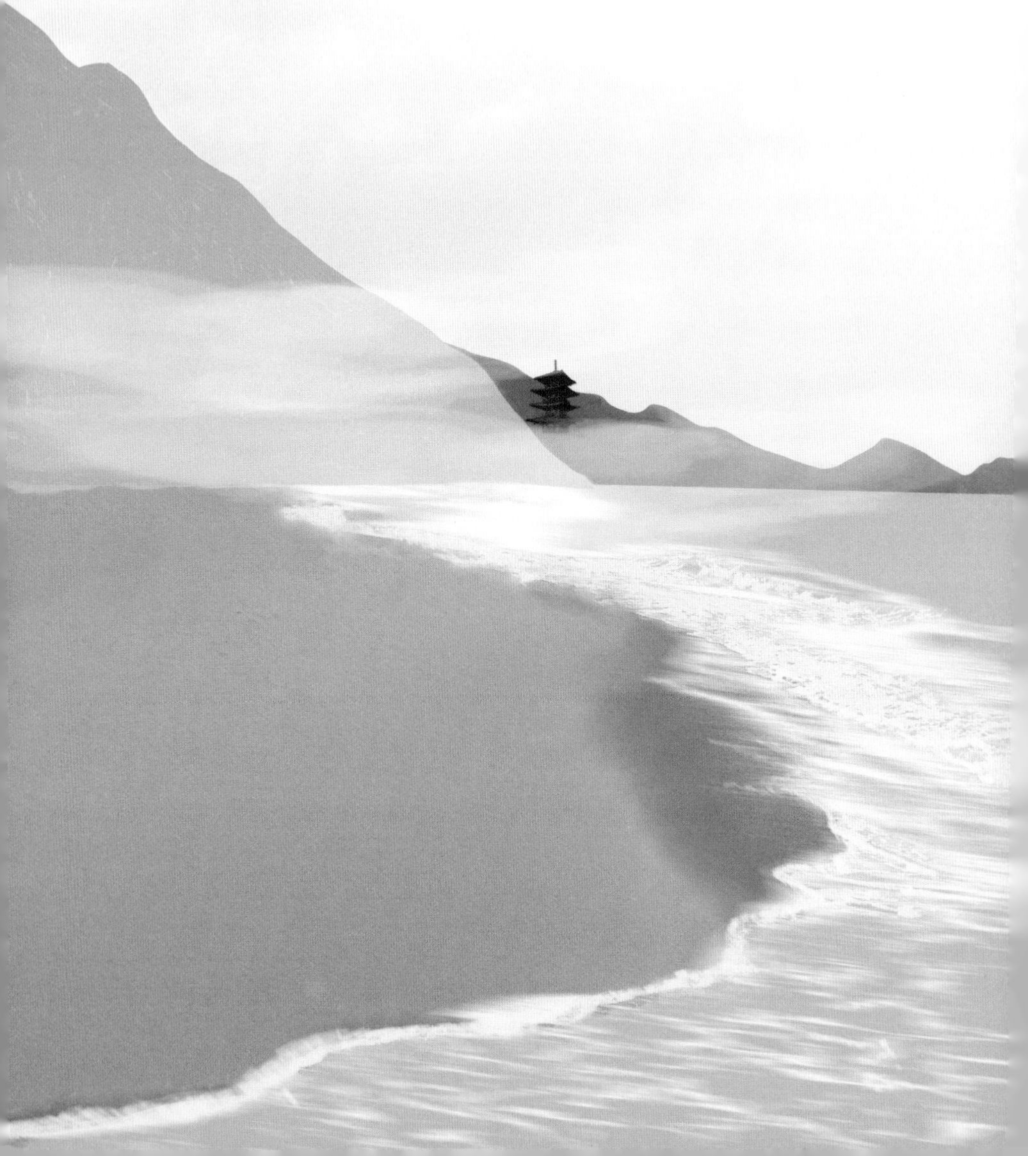

CHAPTER 5
EMOTIONS

Process and balance your emotions
for peace and contentment

'The vitality of all people inevitably comes from their peace of mind. When anxious, you lose this guiding thread. When angry, you lose this basic point.'
NEI-YEH, AROUND 4TH CENTURY BCE

'Control your emotions, or they will control you.'
CHINESE PROVERB

Think back to the last time you had a strong emotion: maybe joy, anger or sadness. As well as the thoughts you had at the time, where did you feel it in your body? People often describe a bad shock as a punch to the gut, or grief as a weight on the chest or stomach. Conversely, the state of your body affects your emotions. You know that when you're ill, it's hard to feel positive.

In Western medicine, it used to be that mind and body were treated separately. But this is changing. Taking a physical approach to mental health has become part of standard treatment: regular exercise, for example, is recommended for mild depression.

What's interesting about Chinese medicine is that it has always rooted the emotional state firmly in the body. So, depression, for example, is described as an imbalance of the organs, almost always involving the liver.

In fact, every emotion we experience is described by Chinese medicine as being housed in the body, each one looked after by a specific organ. And having this specific physical location for emotions will give you a huge shift in perspective; it means you have a place where you can start healing yourself. You may find that thinking about and treating your emotions this way will allow you to process them and so transform how you feel.

YOUR EMOTIONS AND THE ORGANS THEY'RE HOUSED IN

There's another benefit to having an emotion housed in an organ, too. It means your emotions can highlight if you need to treat a particular organ. Taoist master Mantak Chia explains negative emotions as messages that alert us to an imbalance within.

- Anger: liver
- Fear and nervousness: kidneys
- Grief: lungs
- Joy (over-excitement)/anxiety: heart
- Worry: stomach and spleen

As always in Chinese medicine, prevention is better than cure – and knowledge is power. Recognising that you are, for example, an anxious person by nature means you've won half the battle. You can then focus on supporting your stomach, the organ associated with anxiety.

BALANCING YOUR EMOTIONS

The Chinese belief is this: own your emotions and you master your health. It's important to know that not only are you allowed to express the full remit of human emotion, it's actually healthy to do so. Life will bring all kinds of emotional reactions – and that's normal – but you don't want to let one of them take over, because this is not balance. Even a positive emotion, like being happy, is regarded as just one of the emotions. And so rather than always craving constant happiness, we should aspire to feel an even, quiet contentment.

Being too emotional is considered both a waste of valuable qi and to have a detrimental effect on your organs. If you use up too much of your qi, you are risking illness and even shortening your lifespan. This sounds extreme, but it's why the ancient Taoist masters were very big on contentment and quiet living to achieve a long and peaceful life. They referred to living calmly, between the extremes of emotion, as the 'golden mean'.

This is tricky for us in the West, where we are all about strong reactions and emotions, as long as they are positive. We are thrill seekers, rollercoaster riders, happy high chasers. We romanticise the idea of falling deeply in love. All this takes us, culturally, pretty far away from the quiet life suggested by the Taoists. Let's face it, moderation is a lot less sexy than being intense.

We may not be able to always live a life of total calm, but what we can do is express our emotions in a healthy way. That means not suppressing them, but not being at their mercy. Be aware of how you are feeling; the stronger the emotion, the more likely you'll also have associated physical symptoms.

You'd be forgiven for thinking there are mixed messages here. On the one hand, Chinese medicine says 'don't get too emotional', and on the other, 'feel the feelings'. So how can we find that 'golden mean' or balance? The answer is to accept whatever emotion needs to come out as a natural part of life. Expressing it in a controlled way means you won't become overwhelmed.

Being in a balanced emotional state results in free-flowing qi that will do more to support your wellbeing than any green juice. And once you've found your balance, you can go on to do the deeper work on transcending your emotions in the next chapter (see page 134).

How to balance the emotions

You don't need to completely change your life to find balance. Instead, adapt your daily routine with small changes, applied with a wisdom and understanding of why they will work.

You can do these exercises whenever you have a spare minute; in the car, or when you're brushing your teeth. Once you make them a habit, they will come naturally.

HOW TO PROCESS AN EMOTION

OWN THE EMOTION

Recognise your emotion and name it; for example, 'I'm feeling anxious'. Own that you are entitled to feeling like this.

SHIFT THE EMOTION

On a general level, you can do this with laughter, singing and dancing. Or more specifically, use the One-Minute Rescue Breath Ritual technique (see page 38), the Chinese Smiling Breaths technique (see page 52) or the Six Healing Sounds (see page 56) directed at the organ related to the emotion you're feeling. You can also use tapping (see page 29) in the area of that organ.

PRACTISE REGULARLY

This technique may seem very simple, but you do need to do it! If the emotion is one you're experiencing often, practise shifting it every day. Be aware that the emotion will trip you up a few times before you process it fully.

EMOTIONAL FIRST AID

If you've got one emotion that's particularly troubling you, Mantak Chia has this effective emotional release technique.

1. Tell yourself the emotion does not make you a bad person and that you can learn and grow from it.
2. Think about the emotion that's bothering you. Can you pinpoint what triggered it?
3. Now allow yourself to completely give in to that emotion. Magnify it, scream and shout it, feel it all the way down to your toes.
4. Shake. Shake your whole body, really vigorously, for at least a minute. Imagine you are releasing the emotion and expelling it.
5. Take a deep breath and as you breathe out, imagine releasing and breathing out the emotion. Tell it 'You can go now'.
6. Question what the message of the emotion might be. Ask what you can learn from it. This may come to you straight away, or it might spring into your mind weeks later. Write it down – it helps cement the thought in your head and you'll have a record you can go back to and read.

SEVEN EMOTIONAL ENERGY SHIFTERS

These techniques are good for worry as well as when you feel overwhelmed. They help transform uncomfortable or negative feelings.

1. If you are feeling all over the place

In Chinese medicine, speaking scatters your energy and silence is golden for your mind. When you 'save your breath' you also save energy. So, plan some quiet time in to your day.

2. If you feel overwhelmed

Your liver is in charge of the smooth processing of emotion. So give it some support by gently stimulating the liver meridian, allowing your qi to flow more freely. Starting at the ankles, tap up and down the insides of your legs for five minutes. You can do this using a bamboo tapper or, if you don't have one, a hairbrush with rounded bristles.

3. If you feel anxious

You'll never think or worry your way out of a stressful situation, you can only change its energy. Remember, worrying whether something might have happened or may happen in the future won't affect the outcome. The antidote to worry? Shake. (See page 100.)

4. If you can't stop worrying

This is a fantastic acupressure trick for worry and anxiety. Loosely hold your thumb in the palm of the other hand, so your hand is wrapped around the whole of your thumb. Take a few deep breaths. Either hand is fine.

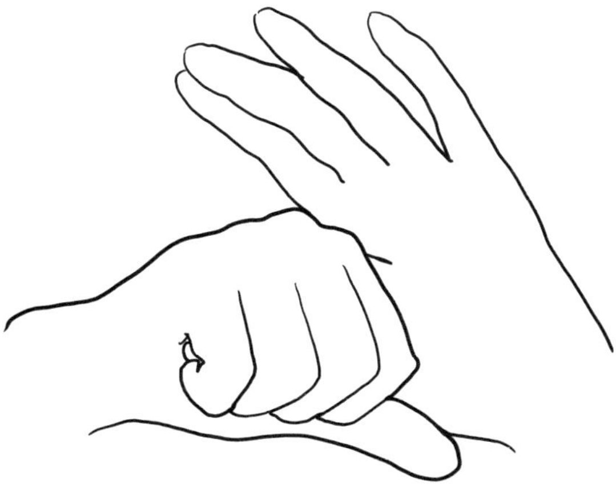

5. If you can't think straight

Breathe in deeply through your nose, then out of your mouth as you do this exercise. The aim is to stretch the scalp with your fingertips.

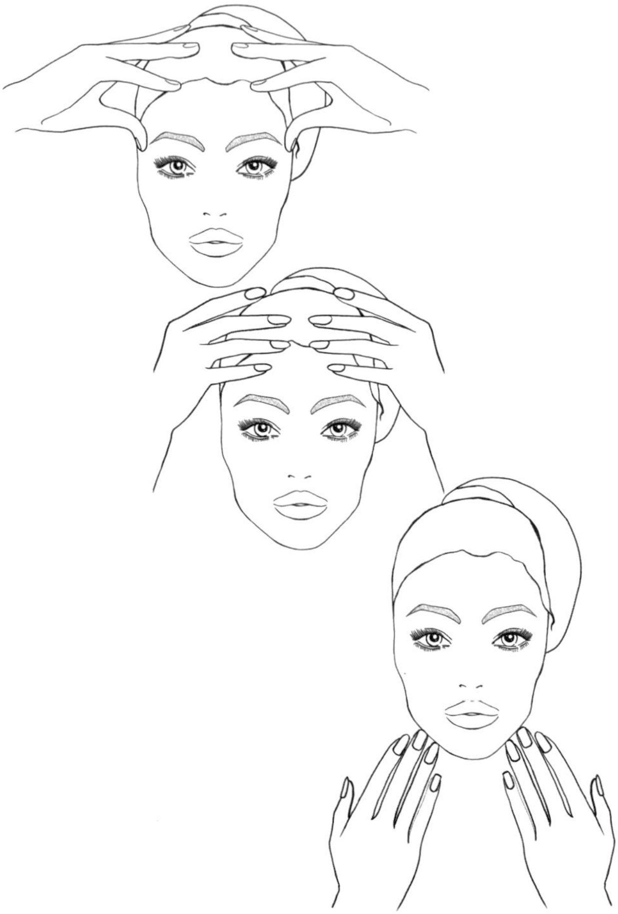

1 Start with your thumbs on the side of your head, each one next to an outer corner of a brow, the rest of your fingertips resting in the middle of your forehead, just above the inner corners of the brow.
2 Apply pressure and slowly pull your fingers apart, stretching the skin, bringing the fingers towards the sides of the head in front of your ears. The thumbs will naturally release as your fingers come towards them.
3 Now bring your fingers back to the centre of the forehead and move your hands a few centimetres up the forehead so your little fingertips are at your hairline. Repeat the stretch.
4 Repeat this pattern over the rest of the scalp, moving the fingertips a few centimetres up and back along the scalp as you go.
5 As your hands move higher up your head they will go behind the ears. When that happens, allow your hands to pull down all the way to your neck and the top of your shoulders.
6 Finish at your shoulders, pushing down into that top muscle (the trapezius) and holding it for a few seconds. Pull across your shoulders towards the front of your throat, hold your hands there until it feels right, then release and drop your hands.
7 Repeat as many times as you wish.

6. If you need a general lift

Make a list of the things you can rely on to bring you joy. I call it the 'I Love List'. Chinese wisdom describes these as strengthening your heart energetically. Yours might be as big and expensive as a massage or take as long as a walk in the woods, but make sure you include lots of small things too. For example, calling your friends, tucking yourself up in bed to read for 20 minutes or enjoying your favourite tea in a particular cup. Then, when you are feeling low, pick one thing to do. Even reading the list will remind you how you can feel. I find that quiet contentment comes from small, regular doses of joy.

7. For grief or sadness

Gua sha loosens blocks caused by negative emotion and restores the free flow of qi. For grief or sadness – housed in your lungs and heart – either tap or gua sha across your chest and up and down your arms, to follow the heart and lung meridians. (See pages 29 and 33.)

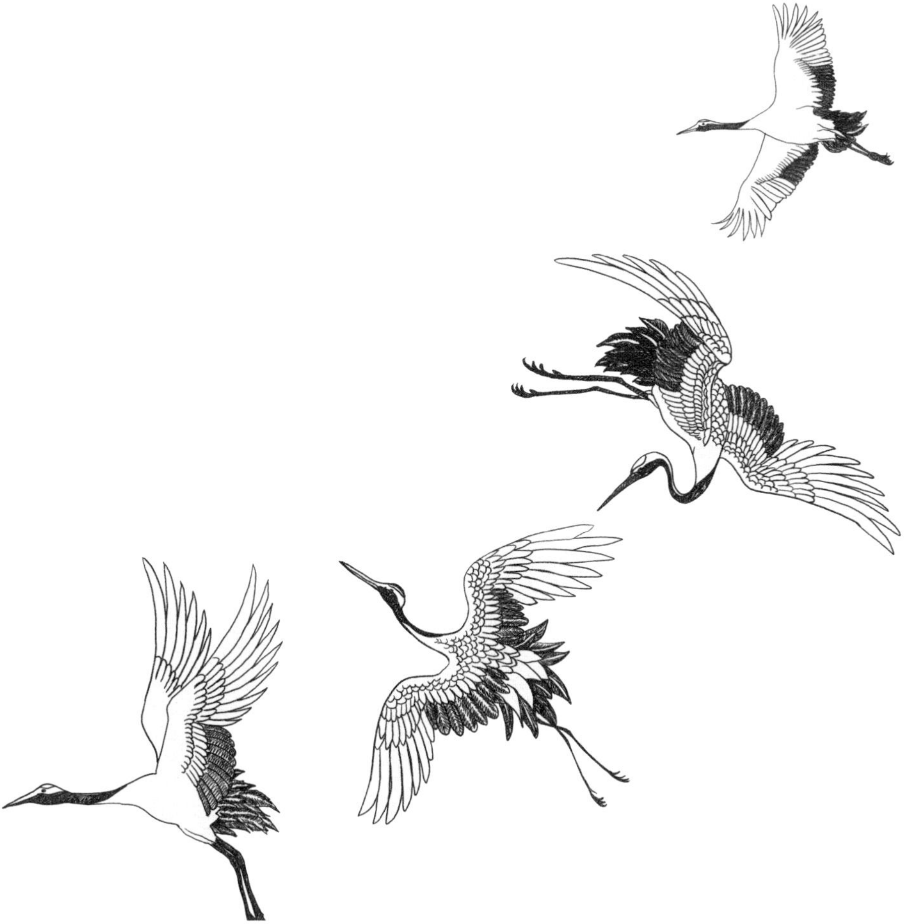

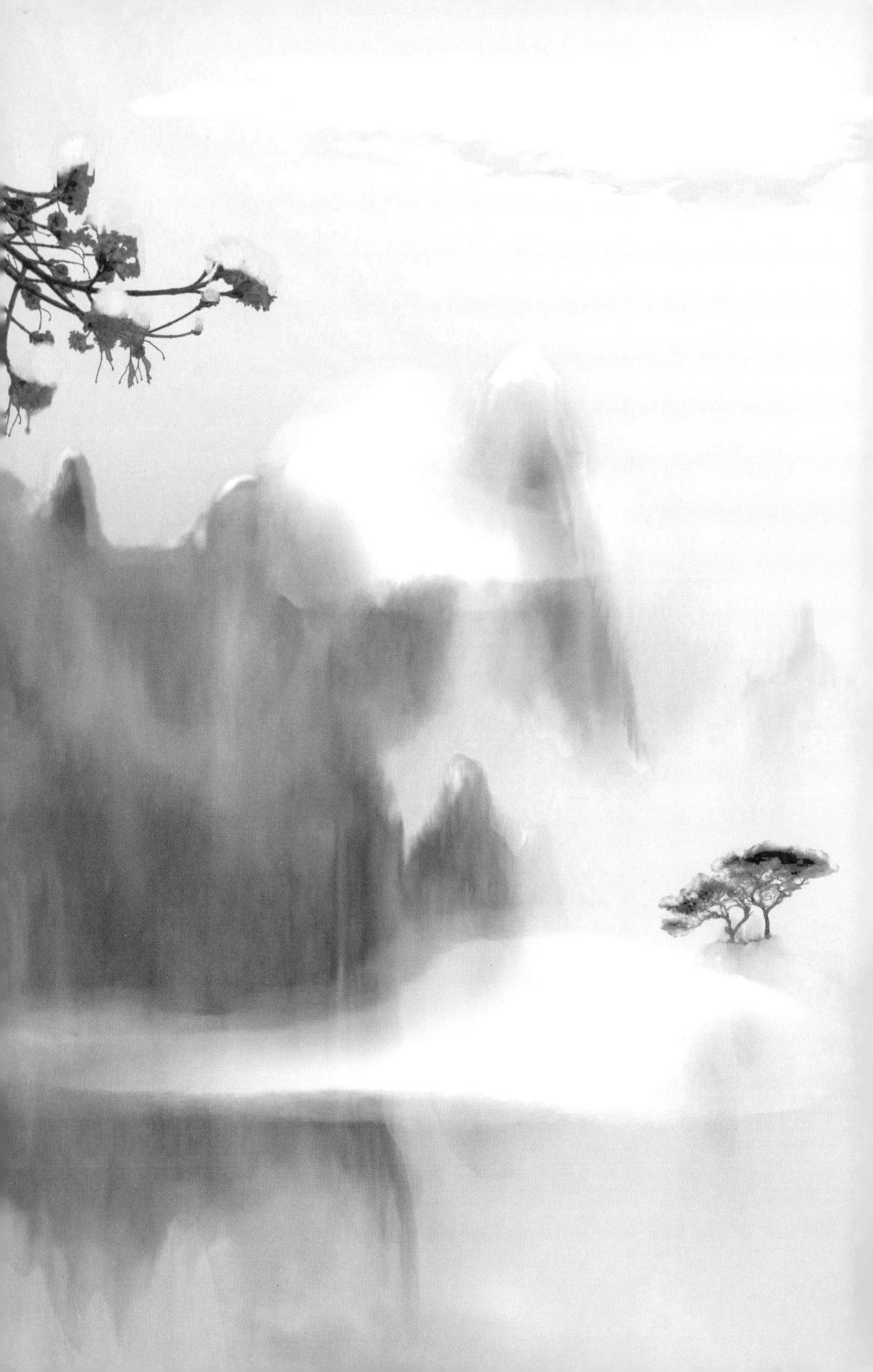

CHAPTER 6

SPIRIT

Live life fully by learning to let go and just be

'If your mind is strong, all difficult things will become easy; if your mind is weak, all easy things will become difficult.' CHINESE PROVERB

'Knowing others is wisdom; knowing the self is enlightenment.' CLASSIC CHINESE TEXT FROM AROUND 400 BCE, TAO TE CHING

How do you define spirituality? If you're religious, you might call it God. If you're not, you might think of it as a search for meaning, a route to personal development or even consider it irrelevant.

Taoism, the philosophical basis of Chinese medicine, takes a very broad view. If you are searching for what spirituality could mean for you, you may find this approach will ring true.

Because it's a philosophy and not a religion, I find the explanations that Taoism gives about the world easy to understand. The Tao (also called the Dao) translates as 'the way' – or you could describe it as the flow of the universe. The idea is that with wisdom and self-acceptance you will align to the laws of nature, to going along with rather than fighting against what makes you, you.

In Taoism, every moment defines the meaning of life. You're not striving towards meaning, you are living it – right here, right now. There is no ultimate goal, purpose or need, nothing to strive for. To live fully, you have to let go and just be. That doesn't mean you don't grow spiritually. In fact, even in old age, as the body is declining, you can still be learning. Isn't that the most positive and inspiring way to look at life?

With this approach, Taoism helps you to live with simplicity and spontaneity as well as to be gentle and flexible. Using simple techniques, you can get back to balance every time your spirit goes out of whack – which, by the way, happens often. Taoism can teach you a calm disposition and how to keep your energy flowing in daily life.

WHAT IS THE SPIRIT?

We all make mistakes – it's an inherently human trait. The Chinese name for the spirit is Shen, or 'heart-mind'. It includes your consciousness and your mind and presence. And according to the Tao, the practise and learning that comes from making mistakes is the route to self-awareness.

Being rooted in Taoism is what makes Chinese medicine is truly holistic, in that it considers all aspects of you as a whole – from the physical and emotional to the spiritual. It says that when you learn to work with your emotions rather than fighting against them (as described in the previous chapter), you also cultivate your spirit and become wiser.

THE ROUTE TO SPIRIT

In Chinese medicine you can heal your body with your spirit and heal your spirit via your body. Taoism says the ultimate way to master emotional balance is via a technique called transcendence. This isn't an out-there meditation or chant, but a practice you can do every single day, which will help you gain spiritual wisdom. When you achieve this, you will quickly feel the benefits of calm and acceptance.

How to transcend emotions

As you can see from the table on page 134 (inspired by internationally renowned classical Chinese medicine expert Lillian Bridges), every emotion not only has an organ, a place where you can work on it physically, but also a corresponding, opposite or healing emotion. To transcend an emotion, you recognise which one you're feeling, then replace it with its healing emotion.

It sounds strange, and it takes a while to master. Every time you cultivate the corresponding, opposite emotion, Chinese medicine believes you are self-healing and growing spiritually. So, cultivating a feeling of compassion is good when you're feeling angry. Having gratitude can counteract feelings of grief.

That said, it's likely you'll yo-yo with how easy you find this – nobody can be perfect, and you don't need to be perfect! It's called spiritual *practice* for a reason...

1 Focus on the emotion you're feeling. For example, you might become aware you feel angry. As you can see from the table, anger is housed in the liver.
2 Next, approach your anger via a physical route. That means taking steps to balance your liver, for example tapping (see page 29) and breathing (see page 28).
3 Now switch your focus to transcending that emotion. For example, you can work to replace irritability or anger with the opposite healing emotions, which in the case of the liver are kindness and compassion.

As I've said – a few times! – Chinese medicine is both holistic and complex, but we can simplify it to create a positive change. With that in mind, this table will give you some basic guidelines and techniques for emotions and the spirit. You may want to see a Chinese medicine practitioner for more specific, personal advice. And if you are struggling with any emotional issues, please do get help from a professional.

Mild symptoms: If you recognise the emotion, but it doesn't significantly impact your life.

More persistent symptoms: If these emotions are affecting your day to day life.

Ideas for healing emotions and spirit

Organ	Harmful emotions	Transcendent healing emotions
KIDNEY	fear, nervousness	wisdom, allowing
LIVER	anger, hate	kindness, compassion, empathy
HEART	anxiety, overexcitement, jealousy, disrespect	unconditional love, reverence
STOMACH	worry, confusion, anxiety (because of overthinking)	contentment
LUNGS	grief, sadness	gratitude, mindfulness

hysical healing actions

OR MILD SYMPTOMS	FOR MORE PERSISTENT SYMPTOMS
est, sleep, listen to calm music, neditate, read, study, enjoy a little weet food.	Garden, grow things, spend time in nature, exercise, go on a hike, drink herbal tea, enjoy a little sour food (see page 181).
hink about the past, think of a sad nemory, volunteer at a charity, listen to he blues, practise a musical instrument, at a little spicy food (see page 181).	Watch a comedy box set, spend time cooking, running, dancing or boxing, hug, do a little sunbathing, eat some bitter food (see page 181).
pend some time with people you dmire, meditate, bathe, swim, learn bout religions or philosophy, clean the ouse, enjoy a little salty food (see age 181).	Listen to calming music, meditate, read, study, enjoy a little sweet food (see page 181).
row things, spend time in nature, xercise, walk, hike, drink herbal tea, njoy a little sour food (see page 181).	Think about the past, think of a sad memory, volunteer at a charity, listen to the blues, practise a musical instrument, eat a little spicy food (see page 181).
atch a comedy box set, spend time ooking, running, dancing or boxing, ug, do a little sun bathing, eat some itter food (see page 181).	Spend some time with people you admire, meditate, bathe, swim, learn about religions or philosophy, clean the house, enjoy a little salty food (see page 181).

THE SPIRITUAL BREATH EXERCISE

Breath is our connection to the divine, according to the Tao. It is in constant motion, and this aligns you to the constant motion of nature and the universe.

In Taoism, there's a particular way to use your breath to engage with your spiritual self: take a deep breath, then exhale slowly and fully. Now pause. Focus on that empty space, where there is nothing in your lungs. This is the moment of the spirit, of complete stillness in the body. Each time you breathe, pay close attention to what you feel in the silence. It can feel uncomfortable to sit with the empty because we are not used to doing it, but you can use this moment to reflect, to be aware of any emotion. Eventually, you will feel peace during the pause.

DAILY SPIRITUAL REBOOTS

If you can, try to do one of the rebalancing exercises below a few times a day.

Set a gong

Set regular (every hour if you can) reboots by programming them into a gong app. When the gong goes, do the spiritual breath while also using this time to reflect and feel any emotion you're struggling with.

One good deed a day

Lao Tzu, a Chinese philosopher and guiding light of Taoism thought to have been alive in the 6th century BCE, said: 'Being deeply loved by another gives you strength, yet loving someone deeply gives you true courage.'

There is an ancient Taoist belief that if you do 3,000 good deeds you will achieve immortality! Though immortality may not be your first concern, consider this: being kind and having a generous will spirit reward you with better physical and mental health and a greater sense of calm, optimism and self-worth. Chinese wisdom states that when you help and genuinely care for others, you will grow spiritually.

Engage with your emotions

As well as assisting with your spiritual growth, engaging with and expressing your emotions makes for a free flow of qi. Every time you think a negative thought, be aware it's a negative thought. It won't stop you having these thoughts, but you will slowly become more actively engaged with your emotional state. Once you've recognised an emotion, you can take steps to transcend it.

Use affirmations

You'll have heard of affirmations as a tool for self-development but you may not know they've been around in Taoism for thousands of years. And for very good reason – they work. There's an ancient Tao observation: 'When you change the way you look at things, the things you look at change'.

Below is a list of suggested affirmations, based on quotes from Lao Tzu:

1 I am content – the whole world belongs to me.

> '*Be content with what you have; rejoice in the way things are. When you realise there is nothing lacking, the whole world belongs to you.*'

2 I am good enough.

'When you are content to be simply yourself and don't compare or compete, everybody will respect you.'

3 I am kind.

'Kindness in words creates confidence. Kindness in thinking creates profoundness. Kindness in giving creates love.'

4 I will let go.

'By letting it go it all gets done. The world is won by those who let it go. The world is beyond the winning.'

5 I embrace change.

'If you realise that all things change, there is nothing you will try to hold on to. If you are not afraid of dying, there is nothing you cannot achieve.'

If you aren't sure about using affirmations, you could try repeating them as an experiment, to see if you note a change in your thought patterns. In fact, disbelief is often the greatest block to how quickly they work. If the ones above don't work for you, you can write your own list of positive thoughts, making sure they ring truc to you. Keep them in the present tense, keep them positive and keep them short.

Practise forgiveness

Forgiveness is regarded as the highest of virtues in Taoism. It's said to heal your pain and elevate your soul. On a more instant level, it makes you feel really good – and strong. The reason is, if you are forgiving, you cannot be angry – and anger is seen as both physically and mentally destructive. To reach forgiveness, first you need to deal with any hurt you may be feeling. A good way to start is by trying to work out why you feel hurt in the first place.

Create a personal altar

As well as shrines in temples, Taoists often have an altar at home too, which serve as a place to connect to the Tao, or to worship ancestors. You can treat yours as a physical reminder to pause and reflect. Or if you want it to be more, it can be your sacred space, which you can use for whatever you need – to grieve, to reflect, to give thanks. What you put on your shrine is also a way for you to express in a tangible way what is happening in your heart. But it doesn't need to be full of stuff – it's enough to have a place where you keep a candle, a plant or fresh flowers.

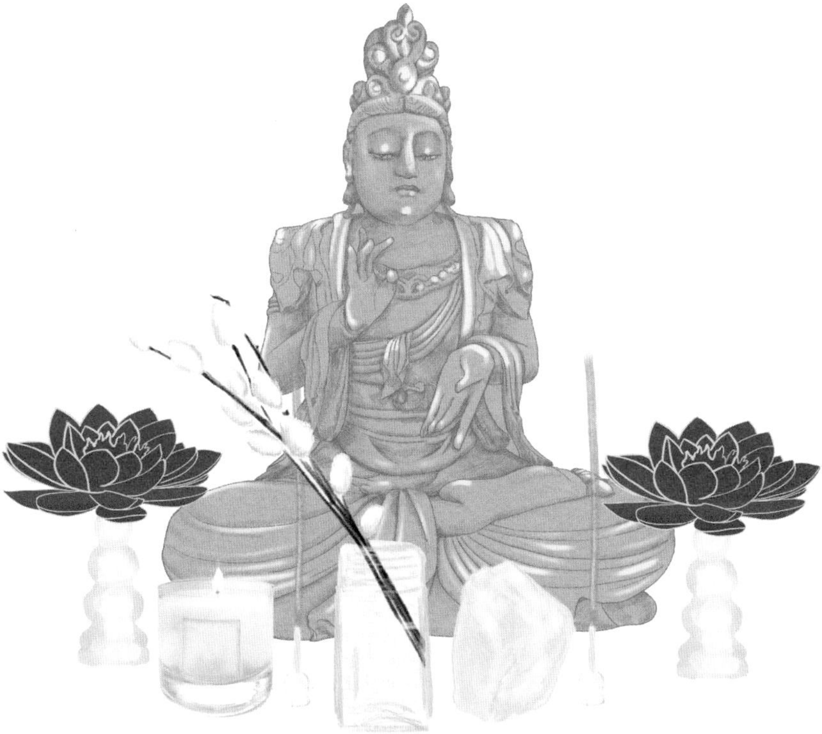

Get some crystals in your life

The use of healing crystals in Taoism dates back over 5,000 years. This makes sense, as Taoism is all about nature. The ancient Taoists believed crystals, minerals and stones could distribute the earth's energy and so help the growth and health of plants, animals and humans. For example, rose quartz tipped acupuncture needles were believed to encourage faster healing. And pearls were traditionally used to cultivate the spirit, by helping the user to relax and become clear about what they want.

However, if you choose only one crystal, I'd recommend jade, traditionally prized in China as more precious than gold. In Chinese medicine, jade is said to clear toxins and balance your yin and yang. You could carry a small stone with you, hold it during meditation or wear it as a pendant.

Be grateful

Regularly say to yourself, 'I'm grateful'. It could be before you eat, before you start your morning qigong practice or after you finish a phone call with your best friend. Gratitude is humbling to your ego. If you don't feel gratitude, Chinese medicine says whatever negative emotion you experience can take hold in the body. In Western studies, expressing gratitude has been shown to alter your brain chemistry, and benefit your mental health. And it costs nothing.

Celebrate your achievements

Give yourself a mental pat on the back. Chinese wisdom sees this as part of developing a sense of worth and self-respect that nurtures you mentally, physically and spiritually. Foster the attitude that you have done good things.

Music and singing

'To cast off worry, there's nothing better than music.'
– Original Tao, 4th century BCE

In Chinese medicine, singing is said to heal and strengthen the spleen and stomach, the organs associated with anxiety and worry. Solo singing is beneficial but singing in a group is even better. In studies, it's been shown to release endorphins and reduce stress levels.

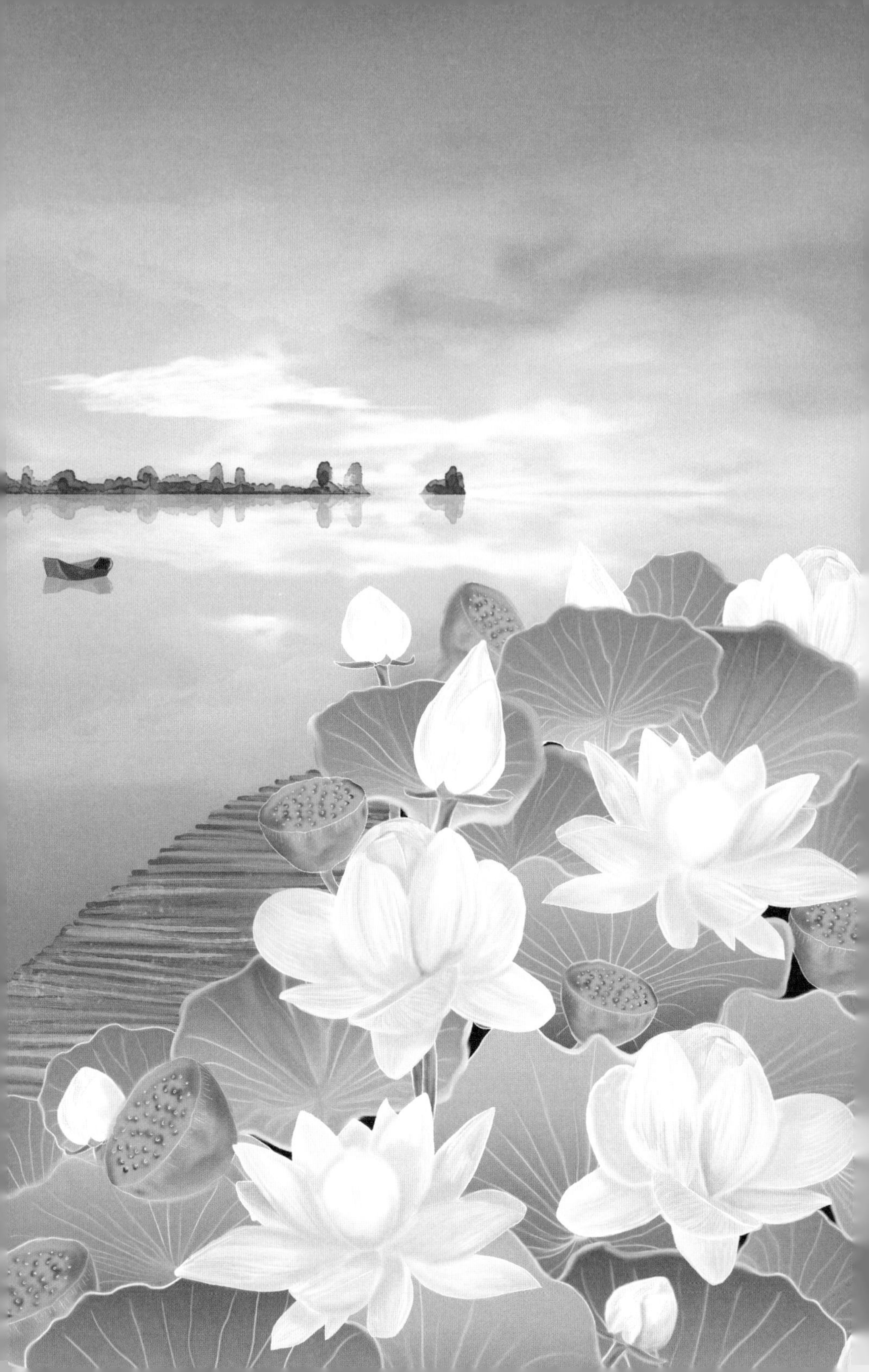

CHAPTER 7

SKIN

Discover how inner health leads to outer beauty

'Beauty is not in the face. Beauty is a light in the heart.'
KHALIL GIBRAN

Beauty, in Chinese wisdom, goes deeper than skin deep. The idea is, focus on your health and beauty will follow. Shiny hair, a healthy weight, glowing skin – in Chinese medicine, these are all signs your organs are happy. Looking after and improving your overall health is one of the biggest investments you can make in your appearance. There isn't the separation of beauty and health that we are used to.

I'm also a great supporter of the Chinese philosophy that beauty isn't just found in the young. The fact that the beauty industry in the West has viewed the signs of ageing as ugly for so long is a world away from the truth. I think the wisdom, experience and contentment that comes with age should be celebrated.

Chinese wisdom says the way you look is a clear indicator of the condition of your overall health, as well as your emotional and spiritual state. A healthy shen, or spirit, produces sparkling eyes because not only is your face a window on your soul, but also on your health. The art of face reading has been an important diagnostic tool in China for millennia.

CHINESE FACIAL ANALYSIS

As face reading is so thorough and detailed, it's a skill that needs to be taught by an expert, such as Lillian Bridges (see page 99). However, there are some basics you can learn to get you started. To begin with, each area of the face has a corresponding internal area. As clear, even skin is a sign of

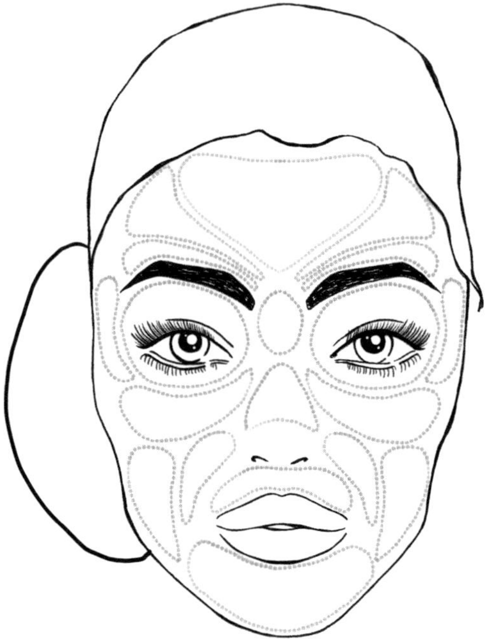

health, any blemishes or changes can indicate specific inner imbalances and stressed areas of the body. It's not as simple as being able to diagnose a disease from someone's face, but you can see clues to health issues. For example, pale cheeks might signpost low qi or a lack of sleep. While Botox might iron out a frown line between the brows, in Chinese face reading, the fact that the line exists at all is a sign your liver may be out of balance.

What is your face telling you?

Skin

INNER AREA: LUNGS

A glowing complexion is reflective of healthy lungs and proper breathing. Open pores, dryness and slowness to heal all signify deficient lung energy.

WHAT YOU CAN DO:

- The One-Minute Rescue Breath Ritual on page 38, ideally outside in clear air.
- Practise the Morning Facial Gua Sha Ritual on page 157.
- For healing of the lungs from an emotional perspective, it's important to learn to accept and appreciate yourself.
- Try the Six Healing Sounds exercise on page 56.

Eyes

INNER AREA: LIVER

If the whites of the eye are clear and just off-white, this reflects a healthy liver. Redness or veiny and dry eyes are a sign of liver inflammation, and blurred vision may be liver deficiency, often caused by tiredness or overuse.

WHAT YOU CAN DO:

- Softly sweep a jade gua sha tool over and around the eyes.
- Eat less very spicy or fat-rich food, drink less caffeine or alcohol. Increase your intake of greens and fragrant herbs such as coriander, parsley and mint.
- Rub your abdomen to stimulate acupressure points around your liver area and support digestion. Start by taking a deep breath then, starting at your navel, use a palm to rub your abdomen in circles clockwise with gentle pressure. Gradually make the circles bigger until you're covering your whole abdomen. Now reverse and rub anticlockwise, in smaller and smaller circles until you are back to your navel. Do 36 times (or as many times as you feel like).

Eyebrows

INNER AREA: LIVER/GALLBLADDER

A vertical line or lines between the eyebrows is a sign of liver stress. Thin or soft eyebrows reflect less liver qi. Shorter eyebrows can mean a gallbladder deficiency and an inability to digest fat. A red skin tone between the eyebrows can means an agitated liver and often anger or frustration.

WHAT YOU CAN DO:

- Gua sha over and in between the eyebrows and over the brow area.
- Support your liver with the suggestions in the Eyes section (see previous page).

Under eyes

INNER: KIDNEYS

Under-eye bags can be a sign of dehydration and/or kidney imbalance.

WHAT YOU CAN DO:

- Make sure you're drinking enough fluids.
- To support your kidneys, rest or, even better, meditate. The optimum time of day to do this for the kidneys is 3pm to 7pm.
- Keep your feet and lower back warm at all times.
- Practise the Turning the Waist exercise (see page 101).
- Massage your Kidney 1 point (see page 84).
- Chinese wisdom says knee rubbing is a simple and effective home remedy for both resolving knee pain and strengthening the kidneys. Take the palms of your hands and rub them on your knees in a clockwise direction 36 times.

Mouth

INNER AREA: SPLEEN/STOMACH

Your lips should be moist, which indicates strong stomach function, while dry lips can mean the opposite.

WHAT YOU CAN DO:

- It's ok to be a little hungry; don't snack between meals unless you really need to.
- Chew slowly, make meals social and eat only when calm and relaxed.
- Sit for 20 minutes after eating.
- People often crave sweets and chocolate because their stomach and spleen are deficient, but this can become a vicious circle, so try to eat less sugar.

Wrinkles

INNER AREA: HEART

The heart is in charge of circulation. Any imbalance in the heart may manifest in wrinkles.

WHAT YOU CAN DO:

- Gua sha your face using a jade tool.
- Gua sha on the chest area will not only assist you emotionally and physically, but should also help calm you, too.
- The heart's key times are 11am to 1pm and 7pm to 11pm. During these hours, try to make some time to relax.

Jaw and chin

INNER AREA: KIDNEYS

A sagging jaw and chin indicates a weakening of the kidneys. In fact, Chinese wisdom this is a classic sign of kidney deficiency that comes as we age.

WHAT YOU CAN DO:

- Gua sha in an upwards motion on your neck and along your jaw line.
- Take the steps to support your kidneys suggested in the Under eyes section.
- Practise the Swimming Dragon exercise on page 104.

AGE BEFORE BEAUTY

You look your most beautiful when your spirit is being expressed, for example when you are talking excitedly about a passion. In Chinese wisdom, the definition of beauty is a face that reflects the shen, or spirit. Skincare and nutrition are important to skin and to ageing well, but the truth is, if you can cultivate your soul to its true beauty, this will then be reflected on your face. And this effect will only improve with age.

Chinese wisdom says there is a specific technique for this kind of beauty, which is to turn everyday emotions into their associated higher or healing emotions, as you learnt in the Spirit chapter (see page 134). So, for example, you turn anger into compassion or fear into wisdom (see table below). The belief is, if the expressions on your face reflect these beautiful emotions, you will be beautiful.

This may sound bizarre to our Western minds. After all, if you are feeling angry, you look angry. The idea is not to deny how you feel, but to transcend the negative emotions. All you have to do, is arrange your face into the healing emotion and intend it. This will reflect in your face as beauty, a look of softness, serenity or warmth.

A couple of these may sound tricky, for example, how do you cultivate wisdom? By learning from your mistakes and tapping into that wisdom, which will then take away fear. The meaning of 'the right course of action', is that you already know the right thing to do, even if it's the harder path to follow. Be certain of this, and it will alleviate your worry which will show in your face.

Emotion you experience	Higher virtue to cultivate	What people will see
Anger	compassion	a look of softness
Fear	wisdom	a look of serenity
Grief	gratitude	a look of rapture
Joy (over excitement)	unconditional love	a glow of warmth
Worry	right course of action	a look of clarity

SKINCARE FROM THE INSIDE

In my opinion, facial gua sha is quite simply the greatest ever gift to skin. Used for millennia by Asian women, I'm so happy it's finally starting to catch on in the West. Thank you, China! So many people have told me, when they make it a daily practice their skin looks its freshest and best.

Gua sha is different from other kinds of massage because you press-stroke the skin using a tool (see page 32). Practise it regularly and it offers myriad amazing benefits, increasing the microcirculation that delivers oxygen and nutrients and removes waste. You can add it to your existing skincare regime alongside your favourite skincare products. I'd even say it can be a natural alternative to Botox, so much so that it's been nicknamed the 'Eastern Facelift'.

A NOTE ON USING A JADE TOOL

You can use a specific jade tool for gua sha (available online), or you can use the edge of a Chinese porcelain soup spoon. Even doing gua sha with a spoon and inexpensive rice bran oil and some deep, considered breathing can be transformative for your skin. But I am a big fan of jade tools because they're shaped to fit your face, with curved points that can be used to activate specific acupressure points and help with flow of qi. And research studies show that, when heated, certified jade radiates healing far infrared rays.

If you do decide to invest in a jade tool, be careful the product you are buying is certified. Cheaper jade tools are often resin, composites or plastic – and not always ethically produced.

MORNING FACIAL GUA SHA RITUAL

This is a super-quick exercise to wake up your face and eradicate all signs of sleep. Take your jade tool into the shower and use the water as a lubricant. Simply press-stroke gently all over your face for about a minute. There's really no right or wrong way, do what feels good. If you do want a basic routine to follow, try this:

1 Press the tool gently all over your neck, face and décolletage.
2 Gently press and hold the tool under each eye, then over each eye, with the lid shut.
3 Starting at the neck, press-stroke down to the base of your throat. This helps move the lymph and gid rid of puffiness.
4 Angling the tool at 45 degrees in the direction that you want to work, use the inner rounded edge to press-stroke the forehead, the cheekbones, then the lips – about eight sweeps in each place. Use the double curved end on your throat and jawline.

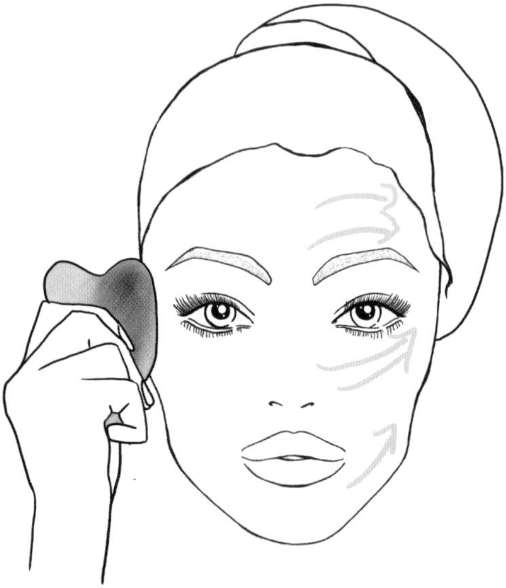

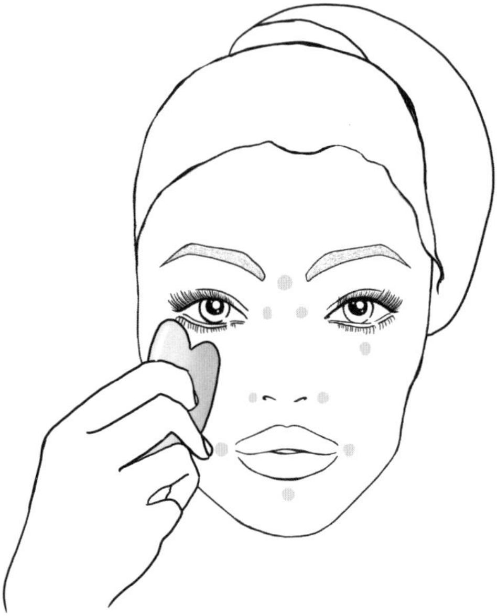

EVENING FACIAL GUA SHA RITUAL

In the evening, indulge yourself with a little more time and attention. Choose any oil that's suitable for your face. If you've got a favourite facial oil, use that, otherwise rice bran oil is a good option. With a scented oil, spend a few seconds deeply inhaling it. Follow the morning technique but spend longer on each section. Really work into any tight areas of your face.

If you have more time, you can use your tool to activate some of the acupressure points on your face. This is a great way to support your organs – and it feels amazing.

1 Using the curved end, press on the outer corners of the lips. This will help tighten the skin.
2 Gently stroking on the sides of the nose helps relieve sinusitis.
3 Using the double edged tip, press on the bridge of your nose and into the corners of your eyes to help release stress and tension and alleviate headaches.
4 Hold the tool flat under the eyes to help reduce eye bags and brighten the eyes.
5 Using the double edged tip, press along the chin to relax the jaw.
6 Pressing the middle of the forehead, between the eyebrows, is great for stress relief.

COMBING THERAPY

This Chinese self-healing treatment involves drawing a very wide-toothed comb, usually made of jade, along the surface of the scalp (see opposite). As long ago as during the Sui Dynasty (581–618 CE), physicians wrote about its multiple health benefits. The theory is, combing stimulates the multiple acupressure points on the head and so the meridians that flow through the scalp.

This ancient technique is ideal for the modern world, in which we spend hours on screens. The restricted blood flow from holding the same position most of the day, as well as stress, can lead to blockages in the meridians of the neck and head. This can cause headaches, eye pain, fatigue, neck and shoulder tension and back pain.

The jade comb stimulates the scalp and circulation, releasing tension so more nutrients can be delivered to the hair follicles. This may be why this technique was traditionally used to support hair growth and treat a dry scalp. You may also find this kind of head massage hugely relaxing!

THE JADE COMB RITUAL

I recommend you comb first thing in the morning to stimulate your scalp and give you a wake-up boost. You can also comb in the evening before bed, to help promote deep and relaxing sleep.

1. There is no need to wet your hair. Start at the frontal hairline and slowly comb backwards, covering all of your head with a light but firm pressure. If you have long hair and it gets caught, shorten your strokes.
2. Then, starting in the middle of your scalp, comb each side of the head down from the crown until you reach the nape of your neck.

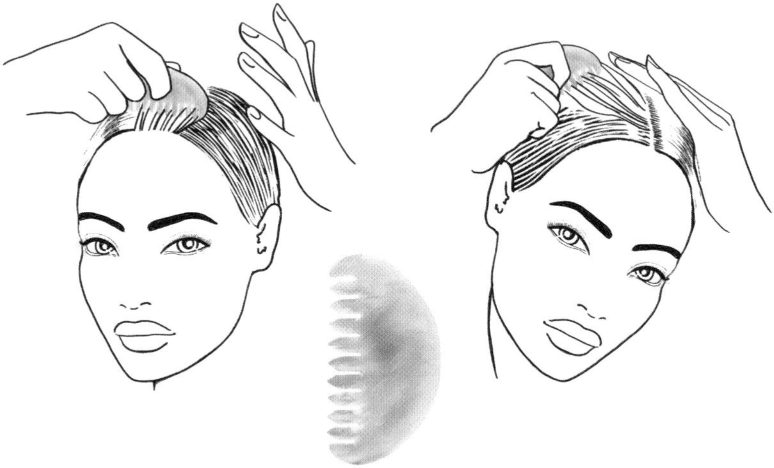

DAILY CHECKLIST

Below is a list of what an ideal day practising yang sheng might look like. You can pick as few or as many yang sheng techniques as you like from this list. Just go with the ones that sound achievable and will make you feel good. Try to be aware of how you are feeling, so you can notice any improvements. When you do, you'll be inspired to do more of these simple practices. Like brushing your teeth, they will become second nature.

Morning routine

In your morning shower do the following:

- Practise the One-Minute Rescue Breath Ritual (see page 38).
- Practise the Morning Facial Gua Sha Ritual (see page 157).

After your shower practise any or all of the following: Tapping (see page 28), Shaking (see page 100) and Lifting the Sky (see page 41).

Daytime routine

- Aim for 10,000 steps a day.
- In addition, try to move around at least once every hour, again using Tapping (page 28), Shaking (see page 100) and also Turning the Waist (see page 101).

These exercises are all really easy and instantly boost your energy levels.

- Try to practise as many as you can of the Seven Daily Qigong Power Exercises (see page 100).
- Sit at a table to eat and take time to enjoy your food. Chew properly and rest afterwards, if possible, to aid digestion.
- Laugh every day (see page 57).
- Repeat your affirmations (see page 138).
- Aim to be appreciative of the little things.
- Repeat the One-Minute Rescue Breath Ritual during moments of stress and to aid digestion (see page 38).

Evening routine

- Have a Mineral Bath (see page 82) or soak your feet (see page 84).
- Practise the Rescue Breath (see page 38) whilst soaking, extending it into a longer meditation.
- Practise the Evening Facial Gua Sha Ritual (see page 159).
- Do body gua sha, focusing on the feet in particular to help make you sleepy (see page 83).
- Comb hair, using a jade comb (see page 161).
- Do the Lifting the Sky exercise to expel excess yang energy (see page 42).

PART 3

SELF-HEALING FOR THE SEASONS

'Nature does not hurry, yet everything is accomplished.'
LAO TZU

Living in harmony with the seasons might sound a little unnecessary in our 24/7 tech-driven world. After all, we don't have to go to bed as soon as it gets dark, nor do we spend autumn taking in the harvest. In fact, very few of us even grow anything we eat. But seasonal living is one of the most important teachings of Chinese medicine. In fact, the reason I've included a whole section on this is because Taoism advocates it as the single most important principle of health and healing.

Think about how the seasons affect you at a physical and mental level: how different do you feel in winter, compared to summer? Maybe in winter you notice you feel like going to bed at 9pm instead of midnight, or ordering soup not salad, or you would far rather hibernate under your duvet when your alarm goes than get up and get going.

Taoism explains these differences like this: each season's start and finish depends on the slow but ever-changing movement of qi in nature and the planet, and this gives each season its own vibration. As we are inherently connected to the environment, our bodies are attuned to that vibration.

The more we mirror nature, says Taoism, the healthier we will be. So, year round, get in tune with nature by looking at what's going on around you. In winter you'll see stillness and hibernation, in spring there will be unfurling and growth. Summer is about relaxing and enjoying the results of your labours – and in autumn there's a slowing, collecting and taking stock. If you change your routine and habits in line with the seasons, you will notice you have more energy, a sense of calm and a feeling of being in control of your life and emotions. Taoists call this state of wellness the 'golden mean'.

You probably already adapt naturally: maybe you love to eat outside on summer evenings or get up earlier. Maybe you have a favourite warming stew you cook in winter. But Chinese wisdom is nothing if not specific; it suggests ways to adjust what we do every season to stay in balance with nature. The amount we sleep, the food we eat and the life choices we make can all be gently tweaked to bring us into line with the natural cycle.

You don't have to make every change in this section – in fact, it would be impossible. Some of the suggestions will sound simple: for example, go to bed late and rise early during summer to get as much daylight as possible. In winter, go to bed early and rise late to conserve your energy, slow down and enjoy peace and stillness. Be assured that the philosophy they are based on is more complex.

Another way to explain why seasonal change is a good idea is because it helps keep your yin and yang energies in balance (see page 22). Warmth, growth, light and movement are yang, whilst coolness, rest, darkness and nourishment are yin. So, spring and summer are yang, autumn and winter are yin.

FOOD AND THE SEASONS

It's now normal to eat mangetout and mango year-round, but if you think about it, doesn't it seem bizarre? To fly food halfway across the world because you fancy a mango? If you try to make most of your food seasonal and local, not only will you lower your carbon footprint but, according to Chinese medicine, you'll also be aligning what is going on inside your body to the ebb and flow of nature. It says our physical and emotional states are greatly influenced by climate and the environment, their rhythm and seasons, and that being in tune with all of those elements is a good thing.

THE GOLDEN RULES OF TAOIST NUTRITION

In Chinese medicine, foods can be divided into five tastes, and they are each recommended for different seasons. You can find a full list of the five tastes and some of their foods on page 181. A Chinese medicine practitioner will usually make a full diagnosis before recommending particular foods to a patient, because foods are specific to your personal make-up and state. However, there are some suggestions that do apply to everyone, below. Some of these may sound strange because they are so different from the Western dialogue about food.

- Eat locally grown foods, as fresh as possible. If you can, grow your own. This will guarantee more qi in food, which is then absorbed by the body.
- Eat more vegetables and eat them in season. This is important because foods absorb different types of qi during the months they are growing.
- Choose organic or chemical-free foods, where you can, to cut down on ingesting chemical fertilisers, pesticides and animal growth drugs. Taoism says that if food isn't grown according to the laws of nature, the quality of the qi in that food is affected.
- Eat less meat, particularly meat that comes from an animal that has been mass farmed.
- Stimulants – including refined sugar and caffeine – are said to cause excessive liver heat, which can make you feel irritable and anxious.

EXERCISE AND THE SEASONS

Your body will be happier if you change up your workout to reflect the seasonal shifts – you may do this already. In spring and summer, for example, it's good to take your workout outside.

As a general rule, split the year into two. From the winter solstice until the summer solstice is the yang cycle of the year. Start this period by doing slow, soft exercise and gradually build up the intensity in the spring. From the summer solstice to the winter solstice is the yin cycle. From midsummer, begin to slow down by including more soft exercise, such as qigong and yoga. By the time the chilly mornings return, you should have made all your workouts gentler. In fact, the Chinese belief is that it can be damaging to the joints and bones to do full-on exercise in autumn and winter.

HEALTH AND THE SEASONS

Remember how we discussed each emotion being connected to an organ (see page 115)? Well, each emotion and its paired organ also connect to a specific season, during which you should focus some extra attention on that relevant organ, to support it while it's 'in charge'. So, for example, in autumn, you need to support your lungs. This could be by practising the organ's healing sound (see page 56) or by taking deep slow breaths, preferably outside in the fresh air, and gua sha on your chest area (see page 83).

Chinese medicine also believes we are in constant interaction with the energies of the environment – called cold, heat, dampness, dryness and wind and collectively known as the five evils – which can have a negative effect on the body. These energies each have their own time of year too (although they can also arise within the body due to imbalances). Lifestyle changes at specific times of the year can counterbalance their effects on the body.

To give you an example, dampness can come from the body being overwhelmed by external damp, such as damp weather or damp-producing foods (or it may be the result of taking antibiotics). The organ affected by dampness is the spleen; you may have symptoms such as water retention or excess phlegm. You might also feel sluggish and have a propensity to gain weight easily, or suffer from greasy, oily skin. If this all sounds pretty

Season	Energy	Emotion	Organ
Winter	cold	fear	kidney
Spring	wind	anger	liver
Summer	heat and dryness	over excitement/ anxiety	heart
Autumn	dampness (beginning) and dryness (end) sadness	sadness	lungs
Last month of each season	dampness	worry	stomach and spleen

complicated, it's because is! This is where a Chinese medicine practitioner comes in, as they're trained to diagnose and treat. But for the purposes of yang sheng and your own self care, you can support the relevant organ in each season (see table, below left) for example by using the Healing Sounds (see page 56).

HOW TO LIVE WITH THE SEASONS

Winter

Up until the winter solstice is the yin part of the year cycle, so this is when you should be in your quietest contemplative state, nurturing yourself with a slow pace, early nights and nourishing warm foods. But what's the reality for most of us? Late bedtimes, excess stress and comfort eating. In Chinese terms, this is a recipe for disaster, getting you out of balance so you end up succumbing to one of the many viruses buzzing around.

Can you find time to get some balance, to rest and repair? Try to carve out quiet moments in your diary for relaxation, even for doing nothing. Meditation is great at any time of the year, but winter lends itself particularly to this kind of stillness.

After the solstice, yang energy starts to rise, so you can slowly start to become more active. But that doesn't mean going all out in a bid to get fit: yang energy shouldn't be overused.

Stay warm: in Chinese medicine, this will help you avoid the evil of cold. Especially, keep your feet and kidneys warm, so wear thick socks and keep your back covered. You can even wrap a scarf around your middle for an extra layer.

Breathing and moving

Avoid sweating excessively during winter. In particular, the contrast between having the heating up high then going out into the freezing cold leads to imbalance. This time of the year is about conserving energy. Take gentle walks in the fresh air and concentrate on dynamic meditation forms such as qigong or yoga.

Digestion

It's bad for the digestion to eat too much cold, raw food in winter. Rather, focus on more warming foods; hearty, savoury soups and stews, whole grains, cabbage and root vegetables and steaming cups of ginger tea. Suggested foods are less sweet and a bit more salty than usual (see table on page 181). For example, miso soup with tofu, cabbage and fresh parsley is perfect for this time of year. The kidneys are the key organ in winter. Nuts and seeds, such as black sesame seeds, walnuts and chestnuts are good for kidney support.

Sleep

Go to bed early, between 9pm and 10pm and wake up late, around 8am. Aim for 8 to 10 hours sleep a night.

Spring

In China, the New Year is a massive, two-week celebration of fireworks, processions, red lanterns for luck and gifts of money in red envelopes. It shifts each year between 21 January and 20 February, because the date depends on the movements of the moon. It's known as Spring Festival because it celebrates the rising in earnest of yang qi – of vitality and life force. Historically this was the start of the new agricultural cycle of sowing, nurturing and harvesting crops.

The evil in this season is wind, which is said to bring agitation and anger, the negative emotions linked with the liver. This makes it a good time to detox, eat well and have a clear out. One way that Chinese people welcome in the new is to buy new clothes and throw away (or recycle) old and unnecessary things.

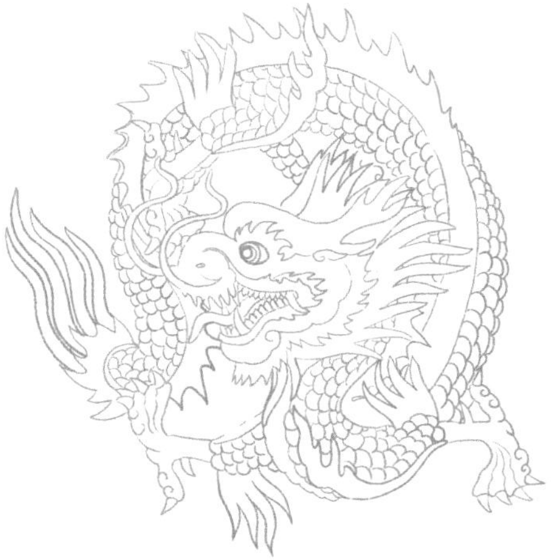

There's also an age-old tradition of deep-cleaning your home before Chinese New Year, to invite in new qi.

Spring is when the rising yang qi becomes obvious, as nature bursts into life. When you go out, you might no longer feel like putting on a thick coat but don't be tempted to shed all your winter layers just yet. You will probably notice you start to have more energy – not only to be active, to get outdoors and do stuff, but also to start new projects. This is a good time of the year to make plans and to think about if you're happy with the direction you're heading in.

Breathing and moving

This is the best time to start or revamp your exercise routine, because it's the season of birth. Chinese medicine divides spring into three months: the first month is good for stretching, paying attention to your joints, limbs, spine and muscles to keep them flexible and moving smoothly.

Digestion

Make sure you drink plenty of fluids now. Try to eat foods that are less pungent and spicy (see table, page 181) and more sour. Lemon in warm water is the perfect way to kick start your morning. It's good to eat some naturally sweet foods in the first month of spring, such as dates or sweet potato. As the weather warms, you can begin to eat more raw food, or food that's been steamed or stir-fried. Roast chicken with lemon served with asparagus is a great spring dish.

Sleep

The advice around sleep in spring isn't quite as strict as in winter, but do try to go to bed early and wake with the sunrise.

Summer

Summer is when the yang energy cycle reaches its peak. Yang is all about outwards energy, which is why you feel like socialising and connecting with people. Summer is the season to celebrate life, and when most of us naturally feel a little more positive. My favourite summer night out involves dancing, dancing and more dancing, which fits well with the advice that you need less sleep now. Try to spend the long evenings outside, especially if you can do it in nature.

Breathing and moving

This is the time to go all out with aerobic exercise, to get really active. But when it gets really hot, try not to overheat – in Chinese terms this introduces the evil heat to the body. This may sound obvious, but it's good to switch to a cooling activity like swimming. And rather than putting your lounger in the sun, Chinese wisdom says it's better to keep cool lying in the shade.

Digestion

Bitter foods will support you this season (see table page 181), including black pepper, avocado, watercress and rocket. You have a green light to eat more raw in summer – salads, fruits, veggies and berries. If you are cooking, steaming or stir-frying is good, the same as in spring. Radishes, tomatoes, cherries, raspberries and strawberries are also great summer foods, ready, ripe and local. During the first month of summer you can have a little salty food. During the second month of summer, limit spicy or pungent food. A good summer salad might include avocado, watercress, rocket and artichoke.

Sleep

To align with nature and the short nights, go to bed later than usual, say 11pm, and wake up early, with the sunrise.

Autumn

The back to school feeling in autumn is summed up beautifully by the approach of organising guru Marie Kondo: 'Keep only those things that speak to your heart. Then take the plunge and discard all the rest.' This is true of possessions, but also of any habits or routines that are wasteful or excessive, or that are linked to a person you no longer are. Your autumn clear-out is about making room for what serves you. Like the trees shed their leaves, it's a good time to shed what you no longer need. You could use your late afternoons and evenings to relax and let go of worries, too. This is a great time of year for learning and self-development.

Breathing and moving

The organ associated with autumn is the lungs, so any exercise that combines deep, mindful breathing with motion works best, from yoga to qigong. You might find the exercises in the Breath chapter (see page 52) helpful. This is a good time of year to do resistance and strength-building exercise too: Pilates or stronger yoga, for example.

Digestion

Begin to eat more hearty, cooked foods as the season goes on. For example, make a chicken casserole with turnips, leeks and onions at the beginning of the autumn, then swap for potatoes and carrots later in the season. Good foods now are nuts, fish and fats, root vegetables, soups and baked foods.

It's also advised to eat strong and spicy flavours – these are the pungent foods. They include onions, cloves, cinnamon, ginger, chilli, basil and rosemary. In the first month of autumn, drink more water and eat some salty foods. In the second month, include some bitter foods, then in the third month, include some sour foods (see table overleaf for foods).

Sleep

Get in the habit of going to bed earlier, between 9pm and 10pm and waking up earlier, between 5am and 7am.

Desk qigong

You could call this the smallest version of qigong! There's a version for each season. Each of your fingers and your thumb has acupuncture points that are connected to a specific organ. So, wiggling that digit will stimulate those points and support that organ. The best time to do this is, of course, during the season when the organ needs the most support.

Simply slowly bend and straighten the digit, for three minutes if possible, whenever you remember.

Season	Season's Key Organ	Finger to Move
Winter	kidney	ring finger
Spring	liver	index finger
Summer	heart	middle finger
Autumn	lung	little finger
Turn of each season	stomach and spleen	thumb

Food types and the seasons

Food type	Good time to eat	Found in
Salt	Winter	Miso, cheese, seaweed, egg, butter, tofu, shellfish, ham, caviar, olives, pickles, tamari, millet, barley, kelp, crab, pork, bacon, mussels, duck, bones, saltwater fish, tinned foods, beef, shellfish, tofu
Sour	Spring	Lemon, sourdough, vinegar, sauerkraut, apple, salami, tomatoes, yoghurt, bread, beef, pickles, pineapple, strawberry, papaya, pear, orange, peach, olives, pomegranate, plum, mango, grapes, fruit juice, mayonnaise, liver, sausage, turkey, sour cream, sprouts, barbecue sauce, beef, chicken, freshwater fish, yeast, asparagus
Bitter	Summer	Black pepper, watercress, dark chocolate, avocado, green vegetables, cauliflower, chicory (endive), rocket, parsley, collards, sesame seeds, coffee, artichoke, broccoli, chocolate, mushrooms, tea, spirulina
Spicy/ pungent	Autumn	Garlic, mustard, horseradish, cinnamon, ginger, mint, vanilla, wine, leeks, onion, wasabi, radish, black bean, coriander (cilantro), turnip, dill, rhubarb, thyme, pepper
Sweet	The last month of each season	Sweet potato, banana, carrots, coconut, almond, kale, oatmeal, milk, honey, beetroot (beets), cooked cabbage, cooked onions, corn, cooked grains, aubergine, fish, goat's milk, prawns (shrimp), walnuts, pumpkin, rice, soy bean, cherry, chestnut, cucumber, wheat

A DAILY TEA PRESCRIPTION

Anyone who has ever visited my clinic will know I always have a pot of tea on the table. There is always a place for tea! It's good to change up your tea for the seasons and according to how you feel.

Spring: Scented teas

Mild and floral, scented teas are refreshing for a gentle, reviving boost after winter. Jasmine is my favourite, but I also like chrysanthemum, rose and goji berry.

Summer: Green teas

Green tea is rich in vitamins, minerals and a calming amino acid called L-Theanine. It's good all year round for anyone who has a tendency to feel hot. Make it with water at 80°C/176°F.

Autumn: Oolong tea

Oolong has been shown to help with weight loss, so it suits this time, when you begin to slow down your activity levels. I also like chrysanthemum tea with honey – it nourishes the lungs and is especially good in the last month of autumn.

Winter: Black teas

Black teas are particularly good if you feel the cold. They help warm the body by improving your digestion and boosting your metabolism. Adding milk is fine if that's how you prefer it.

Mood improver: Rose tea

This enriches the blood and qi, soothing your nerves and lifting your mood. Add dried rose hips or rose petals to boiling water, steep for 20 minutes and drink. Add honey to taste.

Warming/for a cold: Ginger tea

You can add chopped, fresh ginger to any tea. A pinch of black pepper is good when you have a cold, too. If you feel the cold, feel weak or are recovering from illness, ginger powder stirred into hot water is fantastic. You can also add honey.

AFTERWORD

I hope this book will give you achievable, practical and simple ways to transform your health. Yang sheng is a vast subject and part of an even vaster one, Chinese medicine. I'm conscious there's just so much to know – and this is simply a place to start. In this book, I hope I've shown you that you don't need to do everything or know everything. You can just start by building little changes into your daily life.

Once you start adding some of the yang sheng techniques, you will notice a difference. It may be subtle, it may be obvious, but it will be there. My patients tell me they sleep better, or their weight stabilises, or they feel calmer, or have more energy or sex drive. Sometimes, in fact, all of the above! And the more you do, the more changes will happen. But, you don't need to do everything. Remember living with the Tao means calm, quiet contentment – not stressing because you are failing to fit it all in. Do less, 'be' more.

Yang sheng is a way of living to nurture your life. It isn't onerous, it's pleasurable. And because you're giving your body what it needs, it means you can still enjoy a little of what you fancy too. Making life just that bit easier all round.

So please, just use the checklist (page 162) as a basis to keep you on track, rather than following it slavishly. You'll find that after a while, much of it will just become habit. Largely because, like brushing your teeth, it's quick and effective. But, if you can't manage this much every day, don't worry. The rule of thumb I give to all my patients is this: try to look after yourself and those around you. Do that, and you'll be mastering the Chinese art of self-healing.

What I really love to hear are the stories I receive from people who have adopted some or many of the techniques and how this has changed their life too. Please do send me your stories or questions at info@hayoumethod.com. You can also find lots more help, advice and videos on the techniques in this book at www.katiebrindle.com.

FURTHER READING

Once my clients have experienced the power of yang sheng, they invariably ask me where they can find out more. These are just a few of the experts from whom I learn. I urge you to do the same, because they are inspirational:

Master Mantak China, Daniel Reid, Master Zheng Yuan of the UK I Ching Association, Lillian Bridges, my own qigong master, John Munro at Long White Cloud Qigong. Of all the many fascinating books out there, these are the ones I repeatedly recommend:

- *Eight Immortal Healers* – Mantak Chia (2017)
- *The Tao of Detox* – Daniel Reid (2006)
- *Live well, Live Long* – Peter Deadman (2016)
- *Face Reading in Chinese Medicine* – Lillian Bridges (2012)

BIBLIOGRAPHY

INTRODUCTION

Jahnke R, Larkey L, Rogers C, Etnier J, Lin F. (2010) A Comprehensive Review of Health Benefits of Qigong and Tai Chi. *American journal of health promotion: AJHP*.24(6) :e1-e25. DOI:10.4278/ajhp.081013-LIT-248.

Abbott R, Lavretsky H. Tai Chi and Qigong for the Treatment and Prevention of Mental Disorders. *The Psychiatric clinics of North America*. 2013;36(1):109-119. DOI:10.1016/j.psc.2013.01.011.

Johansson M, Hassmén P, Jouper J. (2008) Acute effects of Qigong exercise on mood and anxiety. *International Journal of Stress Management*. 15(2):199–207.

Irwin MR, Olmstead R, Motivala SJ. (2008) Improving Sleep Quality in Older Adults with Moderate Sleep Complaints: A Randomized Controlled Trial of Tai Chi Chih. *Sleep*. 31(7):1001-1008.

Huston JM and Tracey KJ (2011) The pulse of inflammation: heart rate variability, the cholinergic anti-inflammatory pathway and implications for therapy. *Journal of Internal Medicine*, 269: 45-53. DOI:10.1111/j.1365-2796.2010.02321.x

Koopman FA, et al. (2016) Vagus nerve stimulation inhibits cytokine production and attenuates disease severity in rheumatoid arthritis. Proc Natl Acad Sci USA 113:8284–8289.

Irwin MR. (2014) Sleep and inflammation in resilient aging. *Interface Focus*.4(5):20140009. doi:10.1098/rsfs.2014.0009.

Shu-Zhen Wang, Sha Li, Xiao-Yang Xu, Gui-Ping Lin, Li Shao, Yan Zhao, and Ting Huai Wang. (2010) Effect of Slow Abdominal Breathing Combined with Biofeedback on Blood Pressure and Heart Rate Variability in Prehypertension *The Journal of Alternative and Complementary Medicine.*

Jones BM. (2001) Changes in cytokine production in healthy subjects practicing Guolin Qigong : a pilot study. *BMC Complementary and Alternative Medicine*.1:8. DOI:10.1186/1472-6882-1-8.

Ryu H, Jun CD, Lee BS, Choi BM, Kim HM, Chung HT. (1995) Effect of qigong training on proportions of T lymphocyte subsets in human peripheral blood. *The American Journal of Chinese medicine.*

Kok E. Bethany, Coffey A. Kimberly, Cohn A. Michael, Catalino I. Lahnna, Vacharkulksemsuk Tanya, Algoe B. Sara, Brantley Mary, and Fredrickson L. Barbara. (May 6, 2013) How Positive Emotions Build Physical Health: Perceived Positive Social Connections Account for the

Upward Spiral Between Positive Emotions and Vagal Tone. *Psychological Science*
Vol 24, Issue 7, pp. 1123 – 1132
Rancour, Patrice, MS, RN, PMHCNS-BC. (2016) The Emotional Freedom Technique: Finally, a Unifying Theory for the Practice of Holistic Nursing, or Too Good to Be True? *Journal of Holistic Nursing.*
Church D, Feinstein D. (2017) The Manual Stimulation of Acupuncture Points in the Treatment of Post-Traumatic Stress Disorder: A Review of Clinical Emotional Freedom Techniques. *Medical Acupuncture.* 29(4):194-205. DOI:10.1089/acu.2017.1213.
Maloney-Hinds C1, Petrofsky JS, Zimmerman G. (2008) The effect of 30 Hz vs. 50 Hz passive vibration and duration of vibration on skin blood flow in the arm. *Medical Science monitor.*
Nielsen, Arya et al. (2007) The Effect of Gua Sha Treatment on the Microcirculation of Surface Tissue: A Pilot Study in Healthy Subjects *The Journal of Science and Healing, Volume 3, Issue 5, 456 – 466.*
Yuen WM John, Tsang WN William, Tse HM Sonny, Loo TY Wings, Chan Suk-Tak, Wong LY Diana, Chung HY Hilary, Tam KK Jacky, Choi KS Thomas, Chiang CL Vico. (2017) The effects of Gua sha on symptoms and inflammatory biomarkers associated with chronic low back pain: A randomized active-controlled crossover pilot study in elderly, *Complementary Therapies in Medicine, Volume 32.*
Kwong KK, Kloetzer L, Wong KK, et al. (2009) Bioluminescence Imaging of Heme Oxygenase-1 Upregulation in the Gua Sha Procedure. *Journal*

of Visualized Experiments: JoVE. (30):1385. DOI:10.3791/1385.

Chen T, Liu N, Liu J, et al. (2016) Gua Sha, a press-stroke treatment of the skin, boosts the immune response to intradermal vaccination. Heath W, ed. *PeerJ*. 4:e2451. DOI:10.7717/peerj.2451.

Chan Suk-tak, Yuen WM John, Gohel I Mayur-Danny, Chung Chi-ping, Wong Ho-cheong, Kwong K Kenneth. (2011) Guasha-induced hepatoprotection in chronic active hepatitis B: A case study, *Clinica Chimica Acta,* Volume 412, Issues 17–18.

Xia ZW, Zhong WW, Meyrowitz JS and Zhang ZL. (2008) The Role of Heme Oxygenase-1 in T Cell-Mediated Immunity: The All-Encompassing Enzyme, *Current Pharmaceutical Design 14*: 454. DOI:10.2174/138161208783597326.

Braun Maximilian, Schwickert Miriam, Nielsen Arya, Brunnhuber Stefan, Dobos Gustav, Musial Frauke, Lüdtke Rainer, Michalsen Andreas. (March 2011) Effectiveness of Traditional Chinese "Gua Sha" Therapy in Patients with Chronic Neck Pain: A Randomized Controlled Trial, *Pain Medicine*, Volume 12, Issue 3, 1 Pages 362–369.

Kim J, Sung DJ, Lee J. (2017) Therapeutic effectiveness of instrument-assisted soft tissue mobilization for soft tissue injury: mechanisms and practical application. *Journal of Exercise Rehabilitation*. 13(1):12-22. DOI:10.12965/jer.1732824.412.

James D. McFadyen, Zane S. Kaplan, (2015) Platelets Are Not Just for Clots, *Transfusion Medicine Reviews* Volume 29, Issue 2

Evans SS, Repasky EA, Fisher DT. (2015) Fever and the thermal regulation of immunity: the immune system feels the heat. *Nature reviews Immunology*. 15(6):335-349. DOI:10.1038/nri3843.

Wang X, Chatchawan U, Nakmareong S, et al. (2015) Effects of GUASHA on Heart Rate Variability in Healthy Male Volunteers under Normal Condition and Weightlifters after Weightlifting Training Sessions. *Evidence-based Complementary and Alternative Medicine: eCAM*. 2015:268471. DOI:10.1155/2015/268471.

Li X and Qi LJ. (2007) *Journal of Acupuncture and Tuina Science*. Treatment of insomnia with Guasha

Hachul H, Oliveira DS, Bittencourt LRA, Andersen ML, Tufik S. (2014) The beneficial effects of massage therapy for insomnia in postmenopausal women. *Sleep Science*. 7(2):114-116. DOI:10.1016/j.slsci.2014.09.005.

Fan He Yi, Mao Dong Yin, Li Li and Meng Hong. (2018) Whitening function of Chinese traditional medicine formula via laser Doppler technology, Biotechnology & Biotechnological Equipment, DOI: 10.1080/13102818.2017.1413419

Vairo GL, Miller SJ, McBrier NM, Buckley WE. (2009) Systematic Review of Efficacy for Manual Lymphatic Drainage Techniques in Sports Medicine and Rehabilitation: An Evidence-Based Practice Approach. *The Journal of Manual & Manipulative Therapy*. 17(3):e80-e89.

Kim IH, Kim TY, Ko YW. (2016) The effect of a scalp massage on stress hormone, blood pressure, and heart rate of healthy female. *Journal of Physical Therapy Science*. 28(10):2703-2707. DOI:10.1589/jpts.28.2703.

Faulkner SH, Jackson S, Fatania G and Leicht CA. (2017) The effect of passive heating on heat shock protein 70 and interleukin-6: A possible treatment tool for metabolic diseases?, *Temperature*, 4:3, 292-304, DOI: 10.1080/23328940.2017.1288688

Compan V, Baroja-Mazo A, López-Castejón G, Gomez AI, Martínez CM, Angosto D, Pelegrín P. (2012) Cell Volume Regulation Modulates NLRP3 Inflammasome Activation. *Immunity*, *37*(3), 487-500. DOI: 10.1016/j.immuni.2012.06.013.

CHAPTER 1

Yong MS, Lee HY, Lee YS. (2017) Effects of diaphragm breathing exercise and feedback breathing exercise on pulmonary function in healthy adults. *Journal of Physical Therapy Science*. 29(1):85-87. DOI:10.1589/jpts.29.85.

Russo MA, Santarelli DM, O'Rourke D. (2017) The physiological effects of slow breathing in the healthy human. *Breathe*. 13(4):298-309. DOI:10.1183/20734735.009817.

Wolverton BC, et al. (1989) Interior Landscape Plants for Indoor Air Pollution Abatement. Final Report--September 15, 1989. Stennis Space Center, MS: Science and Technology Laboratory, John C. Stennis Space Center, National Aeronautics and Space Administration.

Claudio L. (2011) Planting Healthier Indoor Air. *Environmental Health Perspectives*. 119(10): a426-a427. DOI:10.1289/ehp.119-a426.

Strøm-Tejsen P, Zukowska D, Wargocki P, Wyon DP. (2015) The effects of bedroom air quality on sleep and next-day performance, *The International Journal of Indoor Environment and Health* DOI:10.1111/ina.12254

Prashant Kumar, Skouloudis N Andreas, Bell Margaret, Mar Viana, Carotta M Cristina, Biskos George, Morawska Lidia. (2016) Real time sensors for indoor air monitoring and challenges ahead in deploying them to urban buildings *Science of The Total Environment* DOI: 10.1016/j.scitotenv.2016.04.032

CHAPTER 2

Sutton, EF, Beyl R, Early KS, Cefalu WT, Ravussin E, Peterson CM. (2018) Early Time-Restricted Feeding Improves Insulin Sensitivity, Blood Pressure, and Oxidative Stress Even without Weight Loss in Men with Prediabetes. *Cell Metab. 27*, 1212–1221.

Voigt RM, Forsyth CB, Green SJ, Engen PA, Keshavarzian A (2016) Circadian Rhythm and the Gut Microbiome, *International Review of Neurobiology, Volume 131* DOI:10.1016/bs.irn.2016.07.002

Patterson RE, Laughlin GA, Sears DD, et al. (2015) Intermittent fasting and human metabolic health. *Journal of the Academy of Nutrition and Dietetics.*;115(8):1203-1212. DOI:10.1016/j.jand.2015.02.018.

CHAPTER 3

Buijze GA, Sierevelt IN, van der Heijden BCJM, Dijkgraaf MG, Frings-Dresen MHW. (2016) The Effect of Cold Showering on Health and Work: A Randomized Controlled Trial. van Wouwe J, ed. *PLoS ONE*.;11(9):e0161749. DOI:10.1371/journal.pone.0161749.

Cypess M. Aaron, Sanaz Lehman, Gethin Williams, et al. (2009) Identification and Importance of Brown Adipose Tissue in Adult Humans, *The New England Journal of Medicine* DOI: 10.1056/NEJMoa0810780

Faulkner SH, Jackson S, Fatania G and Leicht CA. (2017) The effect of passive heating on heat shock protein 70 and interleukin-6: A possible treatment tool for metabolic diseases? *Temperature*, 4:3, 292-304, DOI: 10.1080/23328940.2017.1288688

Mooventhan A, Nivethitha L. (2014) Scientific Evidence-Based Effects of Hydrotherapy on Various Systems of the Body. *North American Journal of Medical Sciences* ;6(5):199-209. DOI:10.4103/1947-2714.132935.

Hildenbrand Kasee, Becker E Bruce, Whitcomb Rebekah and Sanders P James. (2010) "Age-Dependent Autonomic Changes Following Immersion in Cool, Neutral, and Warm Water Temperatures," *International Journal of Aquatic Research and Education*: Vol. 4 : No. 2 , Article 4. DOI: 10.25035/ijare.04.02.04

CHAPTER 4

Ran Li, Li Jin, Ping Hong, et al. (2014) The Effect of Baduanjin on Promoting the Physical Fitness and Health of Adults, *Evidence-Based Complementary and Alternative Medicine*, vol. Article ID 784059, 8 pages, 2014. DOI: 10.1155/2014/784059.

Li H, Geib RW. (2013) Exploring the use of five color flow cytometry to examine the effect of acute tai chi practice on pro inflammatory monocyte subtypes *Biomed Sci Instrum.* 49:209–215.

Wang N, Zhang X, Xiang YB, et al. (2013) Associations of Tai Chi, Walking, and Jogging with Mortality in Chinese Men. *American Journal of Epidemiology*. 178(5):791-796. DOI:10.1093/aje/kwt050.

Półrola P, Wilk-Franczuk M, Wilczyński J, et al. (2018) Anti-inflammatory effect on genes expression after four days of Qigong training in peripheral mononuclear blood cells in healthy women. *Annals of Agricultural and Environmental Medicine.* 25(2):329-333. DOI:10.26444/aaem/85208.

Rosado-Pérez Juana, Ortiz Rocío, Santiago-Osorio Edelmiro, and Manuel Mendoza-Núñez Víctor. (2013) Effect of Tai Chi versus Walking on Oxidative Stress in Mexican Older Adults, *Oxidative Medicine and Cellular Longevity,* vol. Article ID 298590, 8 pages, 2013. DOI: 10.1155/2013/298590.

Chang Pei-Shiun et al. (2018) Physical and psychological effects of Qigong exercise in community-dwelling older adults: An exploratory study *Geriatric Nursing*, Volume 39, Issue 1 , 88 – 94

Xu DQ, Li JX, Hong Y. (2006) Effects of long term Tai Chi practice and jogging exercise on muscle strength and endurance in older people. *British Journal of Sports Medicine*. 40(1):50-54. DOI:10.1136/bjsm.2005.019273.

Saint-Maurice PF, Troiano RP, Matthews CE, Kraus WE. (2018) Moderate-to-Vigorous Physical Activity and All-Cause Mortality: Do Bouts Matter? *Journal of the American Heart Association: Cardiovascular and Cerebrovascular Disease*. 7(6):e007678. DOI:10.1161/JAHA.117.007678.

CHAPTER 5

Veenhoven et al. (2008) Healthy happiness: effects of happiness on physical health and the consequences for preventive health care. *Journal of Happiness Studies*, 9 (3): 449 DOI: 10.1007/s10902-006-9042-1

Fredrickson B. (2000) Cultivating Positive Emotions to Optimize Health and Well-Being. *Prevention & Treatment*, 3. DOI: 10.1037/1522-3736.3.1.31a

CHAPTER 6

Algoe B Sara, Way M Baldwin. (2014) Evidence for a role of the oxytocin system, indexed by genetic variation in *CD38*, in the social bonding effects of expressed gratitude, *Social Cognitive and Affective Neuroscience*, Volume 9, Issue 12, Pages 1855–1861, DOI: 10.1093/scan/nst182

Hoge EA, et al. (2013) Loving-kindness meditation practice associated with longer telomeres in women. *Brain Behavior and Immunity*. 32:159.

Algoe B Sara. (2012) Find, remind, and bind: the functions of gratitude in everyday relationships, *Social and Personality Psychology Compass* vol. 6.

Wong Y Joel, Owen Jesse, Gabana T Nicole, Brown W Joshua, McInnis Sydney, Toth Paul and Gilman Lynn. (2018) Does gratitude writing improve the mental health of psychotherapy clients? Evidence from a randomized controlled trial, *Psychotherapy Research*, 28:2, 192-202, DOI: 10.1080/10503307.2016.1169332

Daniel Weinstein, et al. (2016) Singing and social bonding: changes in connectivity and pain threshold as a function of group size, *Evolution and Human Behavior,* Volume 37 , Issue 2 , 152 – 158

Sin NL. (2016) The Protective Role of Positive Well-Being in Cardiovascular Disease: Review of Current Evidence, Mechanisms, and Clinical Implications. *Current cardiology reports*. 18(11):106. DOI:10.1007/s11886-016-0792-z.

Schladt TM, Nordmann GC, Emilius R, Kudielka BM, de Jong TR, Neumann ID. (2017) Choir versus Solo Singing: Effects on Mood, and Salivary Oxytocin and Cortisol Concentrations. *Frontiers in Human Neuroscience*. 11:430. DOI:10.3389/fnhum.2017.00430.

Fancourt Daisy, Williamon Aaron, Carvalho A Livia, Steptoe Andrew, Dow Rosie and Ian Lewis. (2016) Singing modulates mood, stress, cortisol, cytokine and neuropeptide activity in cancer patients and carers *ecancer* 10 631

CHAPTER 7

Kim IH, Kim TY, Ko YW. (2016) The effect of a scalp massage on stress hormone, blood pressure, and heart rate of healthy female. *Journal of Physical Therapy Science*.28(10):2703-2707. DOI:10.1589/jpts.28.2703.

Waits Alexander, et al. (2018) Acupressure effect on sleep quality: A systematic review and meta-analysis *Sleep Medicine Reviews*, Volume 37, 24 - 34

Koyama T, Kobayashi K, Hama T, Murakami K, Ogawa R. (2016) Standardized Scalp Massage Results in Increased Hair Thickness by Inducing Stretching Forces to Dermal Papilla Cells in the Subcutaneous Tissue. *Eplasty*.16: e8.

INDEX

ACKNOWLEDGEMENTS

The wonders and brilliance of yang sheng need to be known by many not a few – and this book is the culmination of that dream. This was no easy journey, and many have dedicated their time and talent to it. I offer my heartfelt gratitude to everyone here:

To my family for your bottomless and invaluable emotional support: Richard, Ines, Fergus, Anouk, Arthur and Joy, Keke and Jermaine and Amanda and Gemma.

To Julia May-Brown for your positive energy and brilliant ability to turn my words into sparkling copy and to Brigid Moss for your clever structuring and your elegant editing.

To Naja Conrad-Hansen for the beautiful illustrations. And to Simon Attfield for helping me express what I could see but couldn't articulate.

To my talented editor Molly Ahuja, patient designer Nicky Barneby and all at Hardie Grant publishers, and to my skilful agent Valeria Huerta for taking a chance on me.

To Jax Hill-Wilson and Victoria Fuller for your belief, passion and guidance – and for being my guard rails.

To the whole Hayo'u team for bringing it all together.

To the incredible people in my life who have contributed in ways too numerous to list: Yvonne, John, Ilana, Martin and Katie, Trevor and Roy, Rachel, Suzie, Kelly, Carla, Maggie, Arron, Ian, Patrick, Lucinda, Clare, Lou, Simone, Parosha, Nancy, Julie, Nick, Cat, Ella and Teresa, to name but a few.

To Anna Murphy, Lisa Armstrong, Sarah Stacey, Gill Sinclair and Alessandra Steinherr for having faith.

To the experts and masters who have directly contributed to my understanding and passion for Chinese medicine: Mantak Chia, Peter Mole, Lilian Bridges and John Munro, Ran Chen and the UK I Ching Association.

To the experts who have contributed indirectly through their teachings, which thankfully are widely available: Jeffrey Yuen, Steven Chang and Peter Deadman, to name but a few.

This wisdom has been passed down by generations of souls who have preserved the beauty and preciousness of the most important gift we can ever have – health. To these ancestors we all owe our heartfelt thanks.

ABOUT THE AUTHOR

Katie Brindle is a UK born Chinese medicine practitioner and founder of the Hayo'u Method, which offers a range of rituals, products and tools. She specialises in offering a combination of detailed diagnosis and self-treatment plans drawing upon Classical Chinese Medicine.

After a car accident that ended her dreams of becoming an opera singer, followed by multiple complications, Katie used yang sheng to solve her own health issues. She is now committed to increasing awareness of this remarkable system of self-healing and encouraging people to master their own health.

Katie has been working in Chinese medicine since 2002. Alongside practising massage and reflexology, she studied TCM and qualified as a Five Elements Chinese medical practitioner, graduating from the UK's Integrated College of Chinese Medicine.

A strong advocate of Western and Chinese medicine working together to create a healthier, happier society, Katie has been featured widely in the UK press and regularly appears in the media.

Katie lives with her family in Somerset.

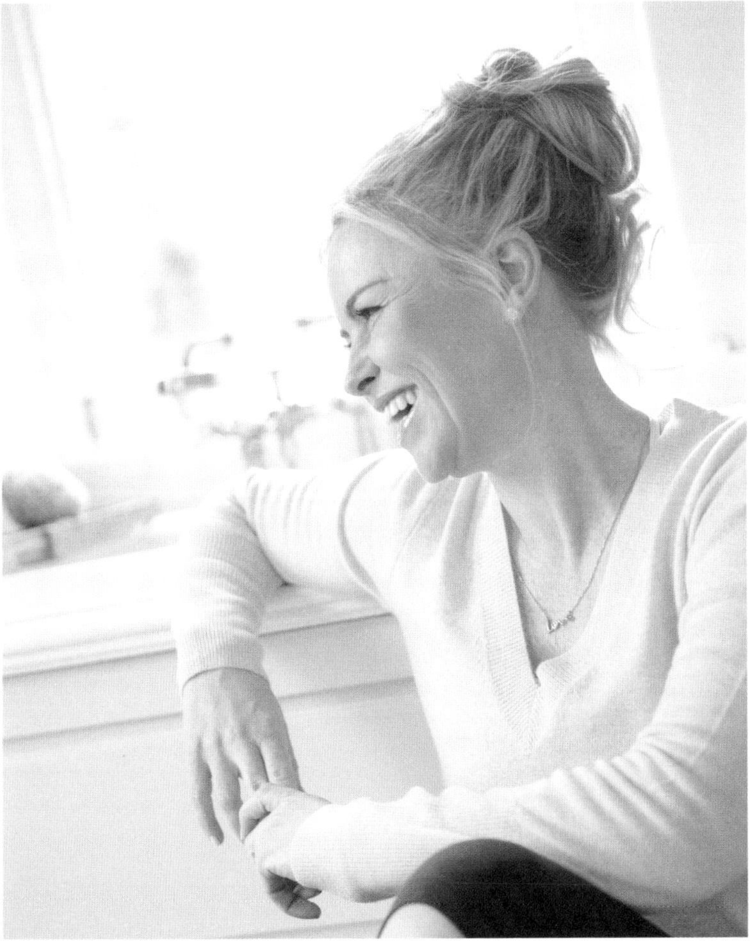

Yang Sheng

Published in 2019 by Hardie Grant Books,
an imprint of Hardie Grant Publishing

Hardie Grant Books (London)
5th & 6th Floors
52–54 Southwark Street
London SE1 1UN

Hardie Grant Books (Melbourne)
Building 1, 658 Church Street
Richmond, Victoria 3121

hardiegrantbooks.com

British Library Cataloguing-in-Publication Data. A catalogue record for this book is available from the British Library.

ISBN: 978-178488-240-2

Publishing Director: Kate Pollard
Senior Editor: Molly Ahuja
Junior Editor: Eila Purvis
Cover and Internal Design: Nicky Barneby
Editor: Helena Caldon
Proofreader: Lisa Pendreigh
Illustrations: Naja Conrad-Hansen
Indexer: Cathy Heath

Colour Reproduction by p2d
Printed and bound in China by Leo Paper Group